Fast Facts

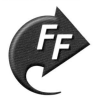

Fast Facts:
Erectile Dysfunction

Fourth edition

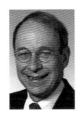

Culley Carson
Rhodes Distinguished Professor and
Chief of Division of Urology
The University of North Carolina
Chapel Hill, North Carolina, USA

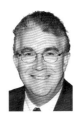

Chris G McMahon MBBS FAChSHM
Associate Professor, University of Sydney and
Director, Australian Centre for Sexual Health
Sydney, Australia

Declaration of Independence
This book is as balanced and as practical as we can make it.
Ideas for improvement are always welcome:
feedback@fastfacts.com

HEALTH PRESS

Fast Facts: Erectile Dysfunction
First published 1997
Second edition 1998; third edition 2002
Fourth edition June 2008

Book orders can be placed by telephone or via the website.
For regional distributors or to order via the website, please go to:
www.fastfacts.com
For telephone orders, please call 01752 202301 (UK), +44 1752 202301 (Europe),
1 800 247 6553 (USA, toll free), +1 419 281 1802 (Americas) or +61 (0)2 9351 6173
(Asia–Pacific).

Fast Facts is a trademark of Health Press Limited.

A CIP record for this title is available from the British Library.

ISBN 978-1-903734-67-4

Carson C (Culley)
Fast Facts: Erectile Dysfunction/
Culley Carson, Chris G McMahon

Medical illustrations by Dee McLean, London, UK.
Typesetting and page layout by Zed, Oxford, UK.
Printed by Latimer Trend & Company Ltd, UK

Text printed with vegetable inks on biodegradable and
recyclable paper manufactured from sustainable forests.

Low
chlorine

Sustainable
forests

Glossary

ACE: angiotensin-converting enzyme

cAMP: cyclic adenosine monophosphate, secondary pathway for corpus cavernosum smooth muscle relaxation

cGMP: cyclic guanosine monophosphate, the second messenger molecule that facilitates the vasodilatation that leads to erection

Corpora cavernosa: paired columns of erectile tissue in the penis

Detumescence: loss of turgidity and erection, usually caused by active sympathetic stimulation

ED: erectile dysfunction

Intracavernosal self-injection: technique in which the patient injects vasoactive drugs into his own corpora cavernosa

MUSE®: medicated urethral system for erection

NAION: non-arteric anterior ischemic optic neuropathy

NO: nitric oxide, a neurotransmitter that produces an erection

NPT: nocturnal penile tumescence

Organic erectile dysfunction: erectile dysfunction caused by the failure of one or more of the essential stages in penile erection, namely the arterial blood supply, venous occlusion or neurological control

PDE5: phosphodiesterase type 5, the substance that breaks down cGMP, resulting in detumescence

PGE_1: prostaglandin E_1, a neurotransmitter resulting in erection

Priapism: a persistent erection that lasts for more than 4 hours

PSA: prostate-specific antigen

Psychogenic erectile dysfunction: erectile dysfunction caused by higher brain center influences in the presence of a normal erectile mechanism

SHBG: sex-hormone-binding globulin

Spinal erection center: an area in the spinal cord through which the spinal erection reflex passes, and which is under neural control from higher brain centers

SSRIs: selective serotonin-reuptake inhibitors

Tumescence: vasodilatation in the corpora cavernosa resulting in erection

Vasoactive agents: drugs that have a dilatory effect on blood vessels

VED: vacuum erection device

Veno-occlusive mechanism: the mechanism by which the venous drainage of the erectile tissues is occluded to allow filling of the lacunar spaces resulting in penile turgidity

VIP: vasoactive intestinal polypeptide – a neurotransmitter in the corpora cavernosa

Introduction

Just 30 years ago, male sexual health was considered to be the exclusive domain of the psychologist. Since then, surgeons have introduced penile prostheses and vacuum devices as mechanical treatments for erectile dysfunction (ED). More recently, basic scientists have determined the physiology of the erectile mechanism, leading to the development of a number of pharmacological treatment alternatives.

This progress has coincided with an increased understanding of the nature of male sexual health problems, and epidemiological data have confirmed that such problems are widely prevalent and the source of considerable morbidity, both for individuals and within relationships. ED is not a necessary part of the aging process, but may occur as a result of a specific illness or as a consequence of the medical treatment of another unrelated illness. Healthcare professionals involved in all aspects of care need to be aware of these risks.

Patients now realize that simple, effective treatments are available and are demanding access to these therapies. The range of healthcare workers involved in the treatment of men with ED continues to expand with specialist nurses, nurse practitioners, primary care physicians and doctors from a variety of secondary care specialties expected to diagnose and treat patients and offer support and advice confidently and confidentially to these individuals. Therefore, it is essential that all healthcare professionals keep apace with developments to provide the best advice about the safety and effectiveness of treatment.

In response to these rapid advances in treatment, several sets of guidelines have been developed to help manage patients with ED. The guidelines include identification, assessment and diagnosis of the condition, modification of risk factors and provision of first- and second-line therapies. This fourth edition of *Fast Facts: Erectile Dysfunction* provides an in-depth view of the overall management of ED and will be valuable to any healthcare professional who encounters men with the condition, particularly as the number of therapeutic options is increasing and patients expect to receive straightforward and effective treatment.

1 Epidemiology and pathophysiology

Epidemiology

Accurate figures for the prevalence of erectile dysfunction (ED) in populations around the world are difficult to obtain. However, data from a number of US and UK studies are similar, so are regarded as the best estimate. The prevalence of complete ED is estimated to be approximately 5% among 40-year-olds, 10% among men in their 60s, 15% among men in their 70s and 30–40% among men in their 80s. From these figures it has been estimated that there may be 20 million men in the USA, and perhaps as many in Europe, who have significant problems with erectile function. It is projected that, by 2025, 322 million men worldwide will have ED.

Prevalence studies show that, when controlling for other factors, increasing age is a strong risk factor for ED, especially after 50 years of age (Figure 1.1). In addition, conditions such as obesity, diabetes, hypertension, hypercholesterolemia and vascular disease – all present in Western populations in epidemic proportions – are causative factors.

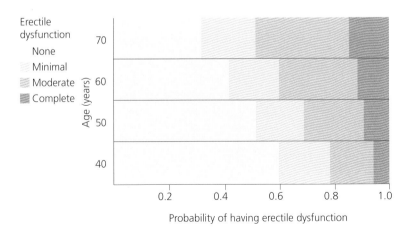

Figure 1.1 Relationship between age and the probability of erectile dysfunction. Data from the Massachusetts Male Aging Study, Feldman et al. 1994.

Endothelial dysfunction appears to be the final common pathway for many cases of ED. Recent studies support the notion that ED may be an early manifestation, and a predictor, of generalized endothelial dysfunction, as well as being a precursor for other forms of cardiovascular disease. Two-thirds of men with hypertension have some degree of ED; 60% of men presenting to an ED clinic had undiagnosed lipid abnormalities. More than half of men with ED who have no cardiac symptoms have an abnormal stress test, and 40% have been found to have significant coronary artery disease when studied. Of men hospitalized for their first myocardial infarction, 64% had ED with onset 3 years or more before infarction. These data strongly support the onset of ED as an early indicator for vascular disease in men. However, the condition remains a source of embarrassment for many men and their doctors and therefore continues to be under-reported, under-recognized and undertreated.

Risk factors for erectile dysfunction. Apart from age, the main risk factors are those for vascular disease (smoking, hypertension, abnormal lipid profile, obesity and lack of exercise). Essentially, any condition that damages endothelial function can result in ED. Other factors include diabetes mellitus and depression (Table 1.1). A study of over 270 000 men with ED showed them to have a higher incidence of hypertension, hyperlipidemia, diabetes and depression.

TABLE 1.1

Prevalence of ED with specific medical conditions

Condition	Prevalence (%)
Overall (age 40–70 years)	10
Severe depression	90
Post myocardial infarction	40
Diabetes	35
Hypertension	25
Cigarette smokers	20

Although the incidence of ED rises significantly with increasing age, recent studies indicate that a large percentage of men remain sexually active into their 70s and beyond; 55–70% of men aged 77–79 years are sexually active, with about six sexual activities per month. However, only half of the men who self-report ED are concerned about it.

It is now recognized that men with benign prostatic hyperplasia (BPH) have a high prevalence of ED. The explanation for this association remains unclear, but it is an interesting observation that may have therapeutic implications. The quality of life of men with BPH is reduced by its effects on sexual function, and this must be considered in patient management decisions.

Neurological risk factors include demyelinating diseases such as multiple sclerosis and any form of pelvic surgery that damages pelvic nerves, such as radical prostatectomy or anterior resection.

Endocrine risk factors include hypogonadism, hyperprolactinemia and hypothyroidism.

Anatomy and physiology of the normal erection

The penis consists of three cylindrical columns of tissue surrounded by a sturdy fascial layer (Buck's fascia), subcutaneous tissue and skin (Figure 1.2). Paired cylinders of erectile tissue, the corpora cavernosa, run

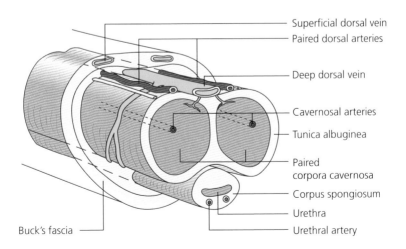

Figure 1.2 Cross-sectional anatomy of the penis.

9

the length of the penis, surrounded by a thick, non-expansile fibrous envelope, the tunica albuginea. Each corporal body communicates with the other through the medial septum that separates them. The erectile tissue itself is composed of a distensible lattice of blood sinusoids surrounded by trabeculae of smooth muscle, which control the sinusoidal blood capacity. The corpus spongiosum of the penis surrounds the urethra and expands to form the sensitive glans penis; it contains similar erectile tissue and is enclosed within the very thin tunica albuginea.

Vascular supply. The arterial blood flow to the penis (Figure 1.3) originates from the internal iliac arteries via the internal pudendal arteries, which terminate as the penile arteries. These divide to form:

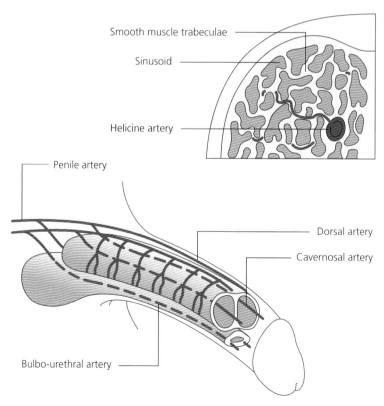

Smooth muscle trabeculae

Sinusoid

Helicine artery

Penile artery

Dorsal artery

Cavernosal artery

Bulbo-urethral artery

Figure 1.3 Arterial blood supply of the penis and corpora cavernosa.

- the dorsal arteries
- the cavernosal arteries, which run down the center of each corpus cavernosum
- the bulbo-urethral arteries, which supply the corpus spongiosum.

Each cavernosal artery gives off numerous branches along its length, called helicine arteries, which supply blood to the sinusoids of the erectile tissue.

Blood from the sinuses is collected by a subtunical plexus of veins from which a series of emissary veins pierce the tunica and join the deep dorsal vein of the penis. The deep dorsal vein runs up the dorsal surface of the penis and joins the periprostatic venous complex (Figure 1.4). Cavernosal veins drain the proximal portions of the corpora.

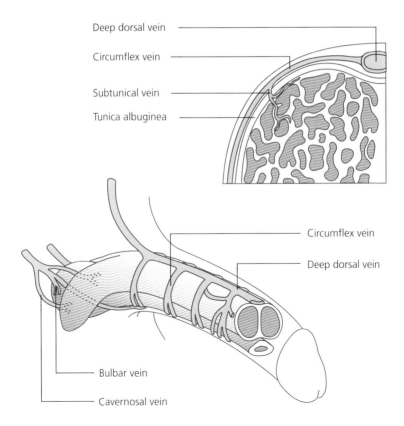

Figure 1.4 Venous drainage of the penis.

Peripheral nerve supply. The mechanism of erection is controlled by the autonomic nervous system. Parasympathetic nerves from S2–4 are the principal mediators of erection, while sympathetic nerves from T11–L2 control ejaculation and detumescence. These autonomic fibers unite in the pelvic plexus to form the cavernous nerves, which run down behind the prostate and into the base of the penis. These nerves and the pelvic plexus itself are susceptible to damage from any form of pelvic surgery.

The pelvic nerves contain sensory and motor elements that form a reflex arc through the spinal cord in an area known as the spinal erection center. A 'reflex' erection therefore occurs as a direct result of stimulation of the penis, and can even occur in patients who have suffered a suprasacral spinal cord transection.

Mechanism of erection

Neuroendocrine messages from the brain (due to either audiovisual stimuli or fantasy) originate in the midbrain at the medial preoptic area, either with or without tactile stimulation of the penis, and activate the autonomic nuclei of the spinal erection center, which send messages to the erectile tissue of the corpora cavernosa via the cavernosal nerves. These messages result in:

- release of nitric oxide (NO) from nerve endings in the corpora cavernosa
- dilatation of the cavernosal and helicine arteries, increasing blood flow into the lacunar spaces
- relaxation of cavernosal smooth muscle, opening the vascular lacunar space
- expansion of the lacunar spaces against the tunica albuginea, compressing the obliquely running subtunical venous plexus, which decreases venous outflow, progressively increases intracavernous pressure and produces a rigid erection; this is the veno-occlusive mechanism (Figure 1.5).

Detumescence. Reversal of these events causes detumescence, driven by increased sympathetic vasoconstrictor activity and the enzymatic breakdown of cyclic guanosine monophosphate (cGMP) by phosphodiesterase type 5 (PDE5). Detumescence occurs naturally

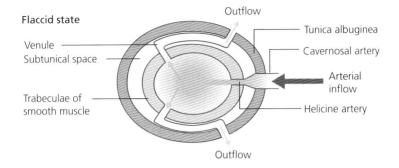

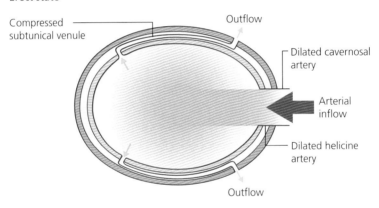

Figure 1.5 The veno-occlusive mechanism depends on compression of the subtunical venules.

after orgasm and ejaculation, both of which are also mediated by the sympathetic nervous system.

Molecular basis of erection

The key modulator of erection is the tone of the smooth muscle walls of the helicine arteries and the trabecular spaces. This is controlled by the level of intracellular calcium in the smooth muscle cells. A number of neurotransmitters and endothelium-derived factors are able to influence intracellular calcium and thereby alter the balance between penile flaccidity and erection (Figure 1.6).

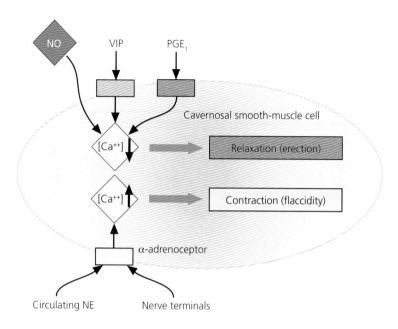

Figure 1.6 Factors that influence balance between erection and flaccidity. NE, norepinephrine (noradrenaline); NO, nitric oxide; PGE$_1$, prostaglandin E$_1$; VIP, vasoactive intestinal polypeptide.

Smooth-muscle relaxation. NO is the most important neurotransmitter in this system. Produced from L-arginine by the enzyme nitric oxide synthase, NO diffuses from nerve endings and endothelial cells into the smooth muscle cells, where it activates a guanylate cyclase second messenger system. Guanylate cyclase converts guanosine triphosphate (GTP) into cyclic guanosine monophosphate (cGMP). This then activates the sodium pump system and opens potassium channels, causing a decrease in intracellular calcium. The effect of cGMP is ended by enzymatic breakdown; the enzyme involved, phosphodiesterase type 5 (PDE5), exists principally in the corpora cavernosa. Parasympathetic nerves containing NO synthase are testosterone dependent, and androgen withdrawal results in increased density and sensitivity of α-adrenoceptors and programmed cell death of cavernous smooth muscle.

Other vasodilator mechanisms exist, including ones involving vasoactive intestinal polypeptide (VIP) and prostaglandin E$_1$ (PGE$_1$), both of which act through the adenylate cyclase system. VIP and PGE_1 molecules stimulate the production of cyclic adenosine monophosphate (cAMP) from adenosine triphosphate (ATP). Like cGMP, cAMP reduces intracellular calcium and thereby induces smooth-muscle relaxation.

Smooth-muscle contraction. The vasoconstrictor norepinephrine (noradrenaline) counterbalances the smooth-muscle relaxation mechanisms. Norepinephrine is released from sympathetic nerve terminals within the corpora, and diffuses across the synaptic gap. It activates α_1-adrenoceptors on the cell membranes of smooth muscle cells. These α_1-adrenoceptors are linked to second messenger pathways that raise intracellular calcium, either by facilitating entry of calcium from the extracellular compartment, or by releasing calcium from intracellular organelles.

A number of other molecules that increase intracellular calcium, such as endothelin-1 and prostaglandin F_2, are also involved in the maintenance of flaccidity. Increased free calcium levels within the smooth muscle cells of the helicine arteries and the trabecular smooth muscle cells activate the contractile mechanism by which actin and myosin molecules slide over each other and form new cross-bridges. Once these are created, a tonic contractile state can be maintained with almost zero energy consumption.

Neural influence

A number of neural pathways to and from the brain influence and sometimes initiate an erectile response. A 'psychogenic' erection occurs as a result of audiovisual stimuli, erotic thoughts or sexual fantasy via signals from the brain to the spinal erection center activating the erectile process (Figure 1.7). However, these pathways can also act to inhibit the same process, giving rise to psychogenic ED.

Several areas in the brain are important in this respect. One is the paraventricular nucleus of the hypothalamus, where dopamine is the key neurotransmitter mediating coordination of neuronal activity. Another, the medial preoptic area, permits sexual stimuli to activate the spinal erection center.

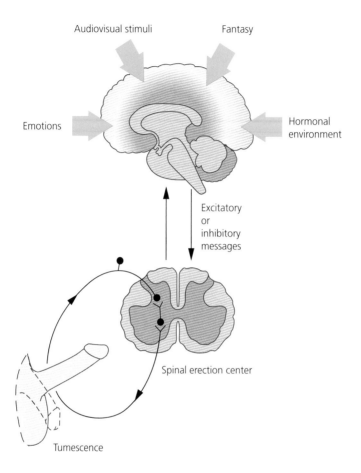

Figure 1.7 Neural pathways that influence the erectile response.

Causes of erectile dysfunction

Modern diagnostic tools have demonstrated that most men with ED have an underlying vascular cause, usually related to endothelial dysfunction. However, there is always a contributing, sometimes substantial, psychogenic component related to performance anxiety; treatment of this component alone may be sufficient to restore normal erections. Other causes of ED (Table 1.2) may lie with changes in the:

- CNS, at the level of either the brain or the spinal cord
- peripheral nervous system, usually due to diabetes mellitus, trauma or surgical injury

TABLE 1.2

Causes of erectile dysfunction

Psychogenic
- Performance anxiety
- Loss of attraction
- Relationship difficulties
- Stress

Psychiatric
- Depression

Neurogenic
- Spinal-cord injury
- Pelvic surgery
- Pelvic radiotherapy
- Multiple sclerosis
- Diabetes mellitus
- Myelodysplasia (spina bifida)
- Intervertebral disc lesion
- Alcohol

Endocrine
- Hormonal deficiency
  - testosterone deficiency
  - raised sex-hormone-binding globulin
  - hyperprolactinemia

Arteriogenic
- Hypertension
- Smoking
- Diabetes mellitus
- Hyperlipidemia
- Peripheral vascular disease
- Metabolic syndrome

Venous
- Functional impairment of the veno-occlusive mechanism

Drugs
- Central and/or direct effect, most commonly
  - antihypertensives
  - antidepressants
  - luteinizing hormone-releasing hormone analogs

These conditions are not mutually exclusive; many cases of erectile dysfunction are multifactorial.

- corpora cavernosa, as in Peyronie's disease
- vascular system – either arterial insufficiency or a disorder of the veno-occlusive mechanism
- endocrine system – reduced testosterone or increased prolactin.

Although it was originally believed that psychogenic problems were the predominant cause of ED, it has now been shown that organic causes are very common, particularly in middle-aged and older men presenting to an ED clinic. In one study, for example, 11% of new patients attending an ED clinic were found to have undiagnosed diabetes and more than half had vascular problems. As described at the start of this chapter, vascular disease may often be the final common pathway in ED.

Key points – epidemiology and pathophysiology

- Approximately 10% of men between 40 and 70 years of age have severe ED.
- Patients with certain medical conditions have an increased risk of ED.
- ED may be a harbinger of future vascular disease and cardiovascular events.
- Multiple neurotransmitters are involved in the mechanism of erectile function; nitric oxide is probably the most important.
- An erection is a vascular event under neurological control.
- All patients have a psychogenic component to their ED, which can be a substantial contributing factor.

Key references

Aytac IA, McKinlay JB, Krane RJ. The likely world increase in erectile dysfunction between 1995 and 2025 and some possible policy consequences. *BJU Int* 1999;84: 50–6.

Fedele D, Coscelli C, Santeusanio F et al. Erectile dysfunction in diabetic subjects in Italy. Gruppo Italiano Studio Deficit Erettile nei Diabetici. *Diabetes Care* 1998;21:1973–7.

Feldman HA, Goldstein I, Hatzichristou DG et al. Impotence and its medical and psychological correlates: results of the Massachusetts Male Aging Study. *J Urol* 1994;151:54–61.

Fournier GR, Juenemann KP, Lue TF, Tanagho EA. Mechanism of venous occlusion during canine penile erection. An anatomic demonstration. *J Urol* 1987;137:163–7.

Jardin A, Wagner G, Khoury S et al., eds. *Erectile Dysfunction*. Plymouth: Health Publication, 2000.

Johannes CB, Araujo AB, Feldman HA et al. Incidence of erectile dysfunction in men 40 to 69 years old. Longitudinal results from the Massachusetts Male Aging Study. *J Urol* 2000;163:460–3.

Kinsey AC, Pomeroy W, Martin C. Age and sexual outlet. In: Kinsey AC, Pomeroy W, Kloner RA, eds. *Heart Disease and Erectile Dysfunction*. Totowa (NJ): Humana Press, 2004.

Lue TF. Erectile dysfunction. *N Engl J Med* 2000;342:1802–13.

Martin C, ed. *Sexual Behavior in the Human Male*. Philadelphia: WB Saunders, 1948:218–62.

Walsh PC, Mostwin JL. Radical prostatectomy and cystoprostatectomy with preservation of potency: results using a new nerve-sparing technique. *Br J Urol* 1984;56:694–7.

A full history and thorough clinical examination of the patient are needed to:
- help elucidate the cause of ED
- determine whether the problem is psychogenic or organic in origin
- identify any clinical signs of the known risk factors.

It should be borne in mind that ED can be an early symptom of a significant systemic condition, such as diabetes mellitus or cardiovascular disease.

Referral to an appropriate physician may be necessary if there is evidence of:
- significant peripheral vascular or cardiac disease
- an organic cause of ED in a young man
- hypogonadism in a young man
- Peyronie's disease
- hyperprolactinemia.

Findings from the history and examination of the patient can be supplemented by investigations to identify the cause of erectile failure. Investigations can be used to:
- confirm the associated underlying condition (e.g. diabetes mellitus)
- give a differential diagnosis of specific causes of ED.

History

A detailed history is probably the most important aspect of the patient assessment. The clinical history has several purposes:
- to confirm that the patient is suffering from ED
- to assess the severity of the condition
- to identify a possible underlying etiology
- to assess the fitness of the patient for resuming sexual activity.

The initial aim, therefore, is to determine whether the problem is one of ED and whether or not this is accompanied by ejaculatory dysfunction, diminished libido or loss of orgasm.

The terminology associated with ED is often confused, and men's expectations of their sexual function may be unrealistic. The severity of the problem can often be assessed by asking simple questions (Table 2.1).

Many doctor/patient consultations about ED are initiated by the doctor. The patient may present with an unrelated problem and only when questioned more closely will he reveal his true concerns. Likewise, there are a number of medical conditions, or 'tickets of entry', that are known to be associated with ED (see Table 1.1 on page 8). Many patients are relieved, indeed pleased, to discuss the problem once the issue has been raised.

Once the degree of ED has been established, enquiries can be made about a possible etiology. The aim of the subsequent discussion is to differentiate between obvious psychological causes and organic causes of the problem. Many men have a combination of causes, however, and the history will contain both organic and psychogenic elements. Topics to cover in discussions with patients include:

- the patient's sexual development and the onset of the problem
- the patient's and his partner's attitude to the problem
- the presence of any obvious stress factors, such as marital problems, financial concerns, sexual inhibitions

TABLE 2.1

Suitable initial questions to ask the patient with ED

- What is the problem with your erections?
- How frequently do you have the problem?
- When did you last have successful sexual intercourse?
- How strong is your desire for sex, now and in the past?
- What has been the effect of your sexual difficulties on your relationship with your partner?
- What is your partner's attitude towards the problem?
- What are you and your partner hoping to gain from any treatments that may be available?

- medical and drug history, in particular smoking, chronic medical illness, pelvic, perineal or penile surgery, pelvic radiotherapy, recreational drug use or psychiatric illness.

The diagnosis of psychogenic and/or organic causes is based on a number of factors.

Psychogenic erectile dysfunction. The association between anxiety and ED should be established. A psychological element should be suspected in a patient who obtains an erection during foreplay or self-stimulation, but fails or fears failure on penetration. In these men, early morning and nocturnal erections are often preserved (Table 2.2).

Psychogenic ED can be caused by a number of problems, principally performance anxiety, but also guilt, depression, relationship problems, or fear and personal anxiety (Figure 2.1). Performance anxiety may be self-perpetuating, with any subsequent attempts at sexual contact being burdened by a 'fear of failure' that only serves to exacerbate the problem. Concerns over whether an adequate and sustainable erection will develop lead to 'spectatoring' (anxious scrutiny of a developing erection), which only serves to inhibit normal sexual responses further. Many men with psychogenic ED may develop a pattern of sexual avoidance due to the frustration and embarrassment of repeated attempts and failure; in turn, this avoidance may be misinterpreted as a lack of sexual desire.

TABLE 2.2

Differential diagnosis of psychogenic and organic ED

Psychogenic	Organic
• Sudden onset	• Gradual onset
• Specific situation	• All circumstances
• Normal nocturnal and early morning erections	• Absent/reduced nocturnal and early morning erections
• Possible relationship problems	• Normal sexual development
• Possible problems during sexual development	

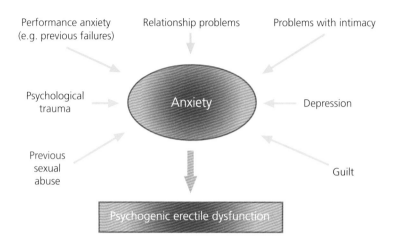

Figure 2.1 Causes of psychogenic erectile dysfunction.

Inhibitory messages from the brain, acting on the spinal erection center, prevent not only the psychogenic erection but also the reflex erection by modulating the normal reflex arc. The inhibitory influence of the brain on erectile function may also be caused by an increased sympathetic outflow and the release of systemic catecholamines, which are known to inhibit the erectile response and cause detumescence (Figure 2.2).

Onset of dysfunction is usually sudden and may relate to a specific occasion or life event. A more detailed psychosexual history, exploring sources of anxiety, guilt, relationship difficulties or depression should be obtained.

Organic erectile dysfunction is characterized by a progressive loss of erectile function with a gradual loss of sustainable erectile rigidity, often combined with the progressive loss of early morning and nocturnal erections (Table 2.2). Many men with ED develop secondary premature ejaculation caused by 'rushed' intercourse to prevent loss of erection.

Several systems have been developed to score the erectile problem objectively. The International Index of Erectile Function (IIEF) has been widely used to quantify the problem. This has been simplified to

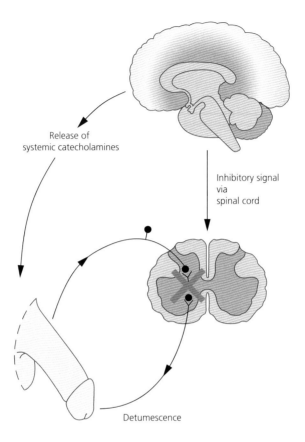

Release of
systemic catecholamines

Inhibitory signal
via
spinal cord

Detumescence

Figure 2.2 The inhibitory influence of the brain on erectile function via the sympathetic nervous system.

five questions, the IIEF-5 or Sexual Health Inventory for Men (SHIM), reproduced in Table 2.3. The scoring system provides a method of measuring a patient's progress from an initial 'benchmark' level.

Concomitant medication. A detailed medical history should be taken to check for the presence of any recognized risk factors. In particular, careful enquiry should be made about current medications, as well as the use of recreational drugs. A number of these may cause or contribute to ED (Table 2.4). For example, antihypertensive agents, such as β-blockers and thiazide diuretics, are associated with ED. In

TABLE 2.3

Sexual health inventory for men (SHIM)

How do you rate your confidence that you could get and keep an erection?

1 (very low) – 5 (very high)

When you had erections with sexual stimulation, how often were your erections hard enough for penetration (entering your partner)?

0 (no sexual activity) – 5 (almost always or always)

During sexual intercourse, how often were you able to maintain your erection after you had penetrated (entered) your partner?

0 (did not attempt intercourse) – 5 (almost always or always)

During sexual intercourse, how difficult was it to maintain your erection to completion of intercourse?

0 (did not attempt intercourse) – 5 (not difficult)

When you attempted sexual intercourse, how often was it satisfactory for you?

0 (did not attempt intercourse) – 5 (almost always or always)

The questionnaire is self-administered by the patient at the initial consultation. A total < 21 indicates ED.

such cases it may be worthwhile changing the patient's medication to an α-adrenoceptor antagonist such as doxazosin or terazosin even though these medications may cause delayed ejaculation or anejaculation. Because of the vasodilatory effects of this class of drug, they may be mildly beneficial in ED, particularly in combination with a phosphodiesterase type 5 (PDE5) inhibitor. Other classes of antihypertensive agents that improve endothelial function and help to preserve or enhance erectile function are:

- calcium-channel blockers
- angiotensin-converting enzyme (ACE) inhibitors
- angiotensin-II receptor blockers.

TABLE 2.4

Medications associated with ED

Major tranquilizers

- Phenothiazines
  (e.g. fluphenazine,
  chlorpromazine, promazine,
  mesoridazine)
- Butyrophenones
  (e.g. haloperidol)
- Thioxanthines
  (e.g. thiothixene,
  chlorprothixene)

Anticholinergics

- Atropine
- Propantheline
- Dimenhydrinate
- Diphenhydramine

Luteinizing hormone-releasing hormone analogs

Antiandrogens

Antihypertensives

- Diuretics (e.g. thiazides,
  spironolactone)
- Vasodilators
  (e.g. hydralazine)
- Central sympatholytics
  (e.g. clonidine)
- β-blockers (e.g.
  propranolol, metoprolol,
  atenolol)
- Angiotensin-converting
  enzyme (ACE) inhibitors
  (e.g. enalapril)
- Calcium-channel blockers
  (e.g. nifedipine)

Antidepressants

- Tricyclics (e.g. nortriptyline,
  amitriptyline, desipramine,
  doxepin)
- Monoamine oxidase
  inhibitors (e.g.
  isocarboazide, phenelzine,
  tranylcypromine, pargyline,
  procarbine)
- Selective serotonin-
  reuptake inhibitors (SSRIs)

Anxiolytics

- Benzodiazepines (e.g.
  chlordiazepoxide,
  diazepam, clorazepate)

Psychotropic drugs

- Alcohol
- Marijuana
- Amphetamines
- Barbiturates
- Nicotine
- Opiates

Miscellaneous

- Cimetidine
- Clofibrate
- Digoxin
- Estrogens
- Indomethacin
- Many others

Erectile dysfunction is a common complication of antidepressant therapy with either monoamine oxidase inhibitors or tricyclic antidepressants.

Selective serotonin reuptake inhibitors may cause both ED and retarded ejaculation.

Physical examination

The examination of a man with ED will be directed, to a certain extent, by knowledge gained from his history. However, it is important to assess the external genitalia, the endocrine and vascular systems, and the prostate gland in most patients (Figure 2.3). The presence, location and size of the testes, together with an assessment of secondary sexual characteristics, will usually be enough to identify obvious hypogonadism.

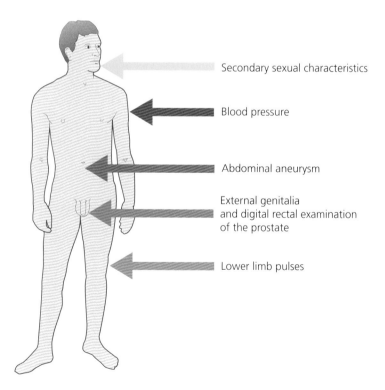

Secondary sexual characteristics

Blood pressure

Abdominal aneurysm

External genitalia
and digital rectal examination
of the prostate

Lower limb pulses

Figure 2.3 Important aspects of the physical examination in men with erectile dysfunction.

Vascular assessment should include measurement of blood pressure, cardiac status and lower extremity pulses; a palpable aortic aneurysm should be sought. The penis should be carefully palpated to exclude the presence of fibrous Peyronie's plaques and to check for phimosis.

The prostate should be the same rubbery consistency as the tip of the nose. Induration or a palpable nodule should raise the suspicion of prostate cancer. Serum levels of prostate-specific antigen (PSA) should be obtained and, if they are elevated in relation to the patient's age and a diagnosis of prostate cancer is likely to be of clinical value, he should be referred for transrectal ultrasound (TRUS)-guided biopsy.

Clinical investigations

The degree to which men should undergo clinical investigation depends on the history of the problem, the experience of the physician and the preferences of the patient. There have been several clinical guidelines published regarding the diagnosis and management of men with ED. Most concur that the investigations performed should address the particular complaints of the individual patient. The investigations can be divided into essential, possible and specialized (Table 2.5). Diabetes mellitus can be excluded by testing the urine and blood for excess glucose. In some circumstances, treatment may then be initiated without further investigation. If this treatment is not successful, referral for specialist advice will probably be required.

General investigations include serum concentrations of total testosterone, fasting glucose, fasting lipids and, in men over 50 years of age, PSA. Further investigations may be required based on the results of these initial investigations including serum concentrations of luteinizing hormone (LH), prolactin, thyroid hormones and HDL/LDL fractions of cholesterol (Table 2.6). Special investigations are not always required, but if patients fail to respond to minimally invasive treatments such investigations may be necessary before other options can be explored.

Specialized investigations need only be performed when a detailed knowledge of the cause of ED is required, and the patient and his partner have expressed an interest in pursuing corrective therapy

TABLE 2.5

Clinical investigations for ED

Essential
- Urine dipstick
- Serum glucose

Possible
- Serum testosterone (total, free and bioavailable)*
- Sex-hormone-binding globulin
- Prolactin
- Creatinine
- Thyroid hormones
- Fasting lipid profile
- Prostate-specific antigen
- Follicle-stimulating hormone/luteinizing hormone

Specialized
- Nocturnal penile tumescence testing
- Color Doppler imaging
- Pharmacocavernosography
- Pharmacoarteriography
- Psychiatric evaluation
- Vascular evaluation
- Cardiac evaluation

*Testosterone levels are best obtained before 10 AM.

or if there is concern about a patient resuming sexual activity. A specialist referral is usually required (Table 2.7).

Color Doppler imaging provides information about penile hemodynamics after maximal smooth-muscle relaxation has been induced with a vasoactive agent. Its aim is to distinguish arterial insufficiency and veno-occlusive dysfunction from other causes of erectile failure.

29

TABLE 2.6

Investigations to identify underlying physiological conditions associated with ED

Investigation	Indication
Prolactin	Low testosterone
PSA	Prostatic symptoms or suspicion of prostate cancer
Lipid profile	Suspicion of peripheral vascular disease

TABLE 2.7

Specific indications for referral to a specialist

- Patient request for specific testing
- Patient requiring vascular, neurological or cardiac evaluation
- Young patient, severe problem
- Patient with Peyronie's disease
- Patient with refractory depression, psychosis or complex psychosexual disorder
- Patients who fail initial therapy

Nocturnal penile tumescence testing. The presence of nocturnal erections, which is used to differentiate psychogenic from organic impotence, can be detected by nocturnal penile tumescence (NPT) testing using devices placed around the penis during sleep. The RigiScan device is designed to be used at home to record the occurrence of nocturnal erections. NPT has a minimal role in the contemporary evaluation of ED, and is usually limited to situations in which potency needs to be confirmed for medical legal reasons.

Pharmacocavernosography can definitively demonstrate failure of the veno-occlusive mechanism to provide adequate venous outflow resistance. This measures the blood flow required to maintain a pharmacologically stimulated erection. Contrast medium injected into

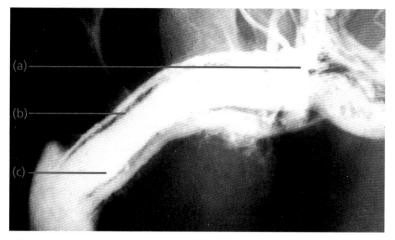

Figure 2.4 Venous leakage is occurring through the dorsal vein and into the retropubic venous plexus during pharmacocavernosography: (a) retropubic venous plexus; (b) dorsal vein; (c) corpus cavernosum.

the corpora will identify the location of any leak, which often originates in the deep dorsal vein of the penis (Figure 2.4), but may also be present in less accessible cavernosal veins.

Pharmacoarteriography. In young men with ED caused by pelvic or perineal trauma, pudendal arteriography before and after a pharmacologically stimulated erection may identify those requiring arterial bypass.

Impact of a diagnosis of ED

It is increasingly recognized that a diagnosis of ED can have a profound impact on a man, his partner and their relationship, his family and ultimately society, as it has a negative effect on the patient's quality of life.

ED can lead to withdrawal from intimacy, avoidance of all physical contact with a partner and an increase in emotional stress, which itself can perpetuate any psychogenic component to the ED. The condition can affect a man's self-esteem and self-image and lead to anxiety and hence depression. Treatment of ED has been shown to lead to resolution of depression and restoration of self-esteem, and thus improvement in quality of life.

Treatment options

The treatment options for men with ED are now varied and effective when compared with those of 20 years ago (Table 2.8). The selection from these various treatment options depends on a number of factors such as severity of ED, underlying cause and patient and partner choice.

However, the fact that ED is associated with endothelial and thus vascular dysfunction should be recognized by physician and patient alike before specific treatments are recommended. If a patient exhibits signs and symptoms of non-psychogenic ED then it is likely that he has an underlying vascular cause, and risk factors should be sought and if possible modified. For example, cigarette smoking and the use of recreational drugs should be discouraged, regular exercise encouraged – it has been shown to preserve erectile function – and depression and dyslipidemias recognized and addressed. If the onset of ED is associated with the introduction of a new drug, such as an antihypertensive, then an alternative agent should be sought (it is believed that α-blockers are less likely to cause ED than other antihypertensives, and may even protect against the onset of ED). These lifestyle changes should be recommended, whatever the cause of the ED, as erectile dysfunction can be an indicator of general well-being.

Accumulating evidence indicates that ED is a predictor of vascular health and thus of the risk of onset of other vascular events such as

TABLE 2.8

Treatment options in psychogenic and organic ED

Psychogenic	Organic
• Psychosexual therapy	• Oral pharmacological agents
• Oral pharmacological agents	• Intraurethral therapy
• Intraurethral therapy	• Intracavernosal therapy
• Intracavernosal therapy	• Vacuum devices
	• Androgen replacement therapy
	• Surgery

hypertension and coronary artery disease. In one study, 20% of men presenting with ED had angiographically silent coronary artery disease. Men with suspected vasculogenic ED should be screened for silent myocardial ischemia by using a treadmill stress ECG. Once a diagnosis is made, the therapeutic options can be put to the patient. They will vary according to the underlying cause, but will probably include oral drug therapy, psychosexual therapy, intracavernosal injections and surgery (Figure 2.5).

Psychogenic erectile dysfunction. Erections are often stimulated by audiovisual stimuli or fantasy; in the same way, however, CNS signals can inhibit the erectile response (see above). Treatment alternatives in this situation include one or both of the following options:

- to identify the source of anxiety, guilt or depression and provide a psychological treatment
- to initiate a physical (drug) treatment that overcomes the specific problem of ED.

Once a patient can obtain an erection 'on demand' from a physical therapy, he may overcome performance anxiety himself.

Psychosexual therapy. Treatment for psychogenic ED cannot be standardized, because the source of anxiety varies between patients. Relationship difficulties, depression, guilt, problems with intimacy and lack of sexual experience may all increase anxiety and/or conflict, which may then manifest as ED.

Psychosexual treatments range from simple sex education through improved partner communication to cognitive and behavioral therapy. The onus is on the counselor to identify the source of anxiety and select an appropriate therapy. Sex education usually involves correction of misinformation and ignorance about normal sexual practice. Improving partner communication may allow partners to overcome their embarrassment about sexual matters and express their sexual needs and desires.

Modern sex therapy owes much to the contribution of Masters and Johnson, who described a treatment program involving a combination of behavioral and psychosexual elements, and reported a 70% success rate after 5 years of follow-up. Today, therapy is more behavior-based and

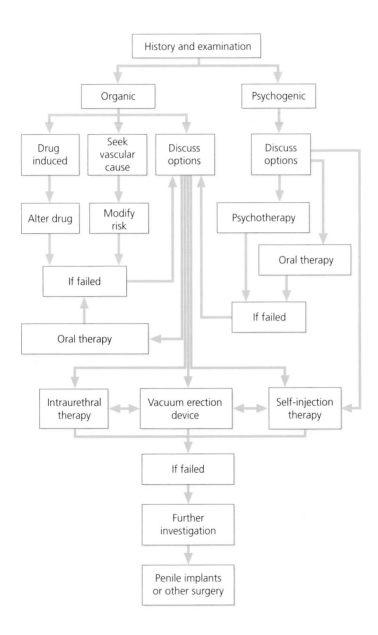

Figure 2.5 Goal-oriented treatment options in the management of ED. It should be remembered that, at any stage, the patient may decide to opt out of therapy and simply accept his condition.

aims to reduce performance anxiety through a programmed relearning of a couple's sexual behavior. Often, this is achieved by gradually increasing a couple's repertoire of sexual activities that do not depend on maintaining a full erection, until full confidence is restored.

The drawback to these types of therapy is that they are expensive in terms of time and resources. They also usually require the presence and cooperation of the sexual partner, though initial individual consultations often help identify relationship problems and expectations. Few long-term studies have assessed the eventual outcomes of these treatments, though there appears to be a substantial recurrence rate after therapy. Many couples, however, derive genuine benefit from this approach, which can also be usefully combined with oral pharmacological therapy.

Physical therapies. Most patients suffering from ED will respond to the safe, effective oral and sublingual pharmacological agents now available. These include the PDE5 inhibitors sildenafil, tadalafil and vardenafil, and apomorphine. Other physical treatments, such as vacuum devices and intracavernosal and intraurethral drugs, are used 'on demand'; however, the rates of discontinuation with these treatment alternatives are high owing to side effects, dislike of needles and unwillingness of the partner to participate.

Intraurethral therapy delivers vasoactive drugs to the corpora cavernosa via the urethral mucosa. The urethra has a rich submucosal blood supply that communicates with the corpora cavernosa through the corpus spongiosum, allowing delivery of vasoactive drugs to the corporal bodies. Therapeutic drug levels can be achieved in men with both psychogenic and organic ED.

Erections can be stimulated pharmacologically using a vasoactive drug injected in to the corpora cavernosa; this intracavernosal therapy can be used to treat psychogenic ED, enabling intercourse to take place, and, with time, may eradicate the 'fear of failure' associated with the condition. Reliance on the drug to produce a satisfactory erection should then diminish, until eventually it is no longer required. These agents may be useful in patients with more severe ED and vascular disease who fail oral agents.

These therapies are covered in detail in the following chapter.

Combined psychogenic/organic erectile dysfunction. A large proportion of patients have a combination of psychogenic and organic ED. Erectile failure resulting from a developing organic problem may provoke the onset of a psychogenic effect once the patient develops the 'fear of failure' on sexual contact. To treat these men holistically, the family physician and psychotherapist may need to collaborate and combine counseling with a physical therapy, such as an oral pharmacological agent.

Organic erectile dysfunction will only respond to physical therapy; however, a contributing psychogenic component, as discussed on page 16, may respond to psychosexual therapy sufficient to restore normal erections. Treatment can be either cause-specific and aim to correct an identifiable abnormality, or general and aim to provide an erectile response regardless of underlying cause. The appropriate treatment option will vary according to the patient's cultural, religious and economic status. Consider:

• ease of administration
• invasiveness
• reversibility
• cost
• mechanism of action
• side effects.

General physical therapies include oral, sublingual, intraurethral and intracavernosal pharmacological agents (described in chapter 3) as well as vacuum devices (chapter 4) and surgery (chapter 5).

Androgen replacement therapy. Male hypogonadism, with testosterone deficiency and ED, can have a number of causes (Table 2.9), and is associated with aging in all men. Regardless of etiology, the aim of androgen replacement therapy is to increase serum testosterone levels to within the normal range, improve sexual desire and function, and maintain secondary sexual characteristics. Although erectile function can be improved or restored in men with marked androgen deficiency, it is less clear whether men with borderline levels obtain any great benefit from testosterone supplementation alone; however, recent studies have shown that PDE5 inhibitors are more effective when

TABLE 2.9

Causes of hypogonadism

Hypergonadotrophic (primary testicular failure)
- Late-onset testicular failure
- Gonadal dysgenesis
- Rudimentary testis syndrome
- Congenital: Klinefelter's syndrome

Hypogonadotrophic (hypothalamic–pituitary dysfunction)
- Pituitary failure
- Prolactin-secreting pituitary adenoma
- Drugs, e.g. luteinizing-hormone-releasing hormone analogs
- Congenital: Kallmann's syndrome
- Prader–Willi syndrome

testosterone levels are normalized. Serum testosterone levels, sexual desire and erectile function all diminish with age, but it is less clear whether testosterone replacement will necessarily result in improved erections, and the precise role of testosterone in erectile function remains controversial. For example, 20% of men undergoing androgen deprivation to treat prostate cancer retain erections sufficient for sexual intercourse. Androgens are known to support both CNS and corpus cavernosum function, with both libido and smooth-muscle relaxation facilitated by testosterone. All hormone substitution therapy aims to achieve physiological serum concentrations of both the hormone and its active metabolites, but current androgen replacement therapies do not always achieve this.

Androgen replacement therapies are described on pages 61–3.

Key points – diagnosis and therapeutic options

- ED is a good index of overall male health, being associated with vascular disease, smoking, diabetes, depression and other conditions. It is the responsibility of the clinician to seek out a possible cause.
- The patient's history is perhaps the most important diagnostic tool.
- Patient investigations are tailored to the history, examination and suspected cause of ED.
- Modification of risk factors should be recommended to men with ED (as advice on overall male health) but rarely leads to restoration of sexual function.
- Partner communication is an important aspect of sexual function and therefore dysfunction.
- Psychogenic ED has a multitude of causes.
- Psychogenic ED may respond to psychosexual or physical therapy; organic ED responds only to physical therapies.

Key references

Barnes P. Sex therapy and erectile dysfunction. In: Carson CC, Kirby RS, Goldstein I, eds. *Textbook of Erectile Dysfunction.* Oxford: Isis Medical Media, 1999.

Cappelleri JC, Rosen RC, Smith MD et al. Diagnostic evaluation of the erectile function domain of the International Index of Erectile Function. *Urology* 1999;54:346–51.

Chun J, Carson CC. Physician–patient dialogue in clinical evaluation of erectile dysfunction. *Urol Clin North Am* 2001;28:249–58.

Kirby M, Jackson G, Betteridge J, Friedli K. Is erectile dysfunction a marker for cardiovascular disease? *Int J Clin Pract* 2001;55:614–18.

Kirby RS. Impotence: diagnosis and management of male erectile dysfunction. *BMJ* 1994;308:957–61.

Kloner RA, Mullin SH, Shook T et al. Erectile dysfunction in the cardiac patient: how common and should we treat? *J Urol* 2003;170: S46–50.

Lue TF. Erectile dysfunction. *N Engl J Med* 2000;342:1802–13.

Morales A, Heaton JP, Carson CC. Andropause: a misnomer for a true clinical entity. *J Urol* 2000;163: 705–12.

Nehra A. Selecting therapy for maintaining sexual function in patients with benign prostatic hyperplasia. *BJU Int* 2005;96: 237–43.

Process of Care Panel. Position Paper: The process of care model for evaluation and treatment of erectile dysfunction. *Int J Impot Res* 1999; 11:59–74.

Rosen R, Altwein J, Boyle P et al. Lower urinary tract symptoms and male sexual dysfunction; the multinational survey of the aging male (MSAM-7). *Eur Urol* 2003; 44:637–49.

Seftel AD, Sun P, Swindle R. The prevalence of hypertension, hyperlipidemia, diabetes mellitus and depression in men with erectile dysfunction. *J Urol* 2004;171: 2341–5.

3 Pharmacological treatment

During the early 1980s, it was established that drugs that relax cavernosal smooth muscle and/or reduce adrenergic sympathetic tone to the penile vasculature induce an erection if administered locally in adequate concentrations. The effects of papaverine, which is a powerful smooth-muscle relaxant, were discovered after inadvertent intracavernosal injection during a surgical procedure. Similar physiological and clinical observations led to a number of drugs being studied as potential therapeutic agents for ED (Table 3.1). Principal among these were the phosphodiesterase type 5 (PDE5) inhibitor drugs, which have become the mainstay of therapy for the majority of patients with ED. This class of drug was first looked at a number of years ago as a possible treatment for coronary artery disease. As a result of the associated effects of the drugs, the mechanism of erectile function was

TABLE 3.1

Drugs with therapeutic potential in ED

Mechanism of action	Drug
Smooth-muscle relaxation	Papaverine
	Nitroglycerine
	Verapamil
	Vasoactive intestinal polypeptide
	Alprostadil
α-adrenoceptor blockade	Phentolamine
	Phenoxybenzamine
	Yohimbine
	Moxisylyte
Phosphodiesterase type 5 inhibition	Sildenafil
	Vardenafil
	Tadalafil
Central nervous system activity	Apomorphine
	Melanocortin receptor agonist

investigated further, and the PDE5 inhibitors were launched as therapeutic options for men with ED, commencing with sildenafil in 1998.

Oral pharmacological agents

Phosphodiesterase type 5 inhibitors are a breakthrough therapy in the treatment of ED (Table 3.2). Nitric oxide, the key neurotransmitter involved in relaxation of corpus cavernosal smooth muscle, acts through a second messenger system involving guanylate cyclase. The cyclic guanosine monophosphate (cGMP) produced is normally broken down by PDE5, a cGMP-specific isoenzyme (see page 14), which exists principally in the corpora cavernosa. The PDE5 inhibitors selectively inhibit this enzyme and therefore potentiate the pro-erectile effect by enhancing the normal vasodilatory erectile mechanisms; sildenafil, tadalafil and vardenafil thus increase the amount of cGMP available for smooth-muscle relaxation and therefore vasodilation and erection (Figure 3.1). They work in response to sexual stimulation to improve erectile function and are thus called 'enhancers'.

These drugs have become the first line of treatment for the majority of men with ED. Three agents are currently licensed for use: sildenafil, tadalafil and vardenafil. These drugs vary little in their overall efficacy in terms of erectile response, but differences in their pharmacokinetics do lead to some variations in drug behavior. The drugs have a slightly different selectivity for the PDE5 isoenzyme and variable inhibition of the other PDE enzymes, and thus have a slightly different side-effect

TABLE 3.2

PDE5 inhibitors are effective for most cases of ED

- Produce a natural erectile response to sexual stimulation by enhancing the relaxant effect of nitric oxide on the corpora cavernosa
- Effective treatment of ED with broad-spectrum etiology
- No evidence of tachyphylaxis or drug tolerance
- Side effects are predictable, well-tolerated and dose-dependent

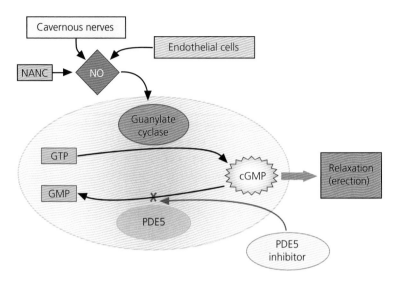

Figure 3.1 Phosphodiesterase type 5 (PDE5) inhibition prevents cyclic guanosine monophosphate (cGMP) breakdown and thereby enhances the normal erectile response. GTP, guanosine triphosphate; NANC, non-adrenergic–non-cholinergic neurons; NO, nitric oxide.

profile. However, the main and most common side effects are related to inhibition of PDE5 and are thus common to all the drugs.

PDE5 inhibitors are cleared predominantly by cytochrome P450 isozymes in the liver. Cytochrome P450 inhibitors, such as cimetidine, ketoconazole and erythromycin, result in reduced clearance of PDE5 inhibitors, thus increasing their plasma concentration and duration of action, but this is not usually associated with an increase in adverse events in patients taking this type of medication.

PDE5 inhibitors have peripheral vasodilatory properties, resulting in modest, and usually asymptomatic, decreases in blood pressure in some patients. Consistent with their known effects on the nitric oxide/cGMP pathway, PDE5 inhibitors are contraindicated in patients using nitrates (e.g. glyceryl trinitrate, isosorbide) or nitric oxide donors (e.g. sodium nitroprusside), in any form, because of the substantial risk of sudden profound drops in systolic blood pressure.

Because of the contraindication of PDE5 inhibitors in patients using nitrates, concern has arisen about prescribing PDE5 inhibitors in patients with heart disease. There is currently no evidence of any direct deleterious effect on myocardium. In randomized studies with sildenafil, the incidence of significant cardiac events has been the same in both the placebo and sildenafil groups. An increasing body of evidence supports the concept that PDE5 inhibitors improve endothelial function and, therefore, are likely to be cardioprotective. Sexual intercourse itself is a minor risk factor for myocardial infarction and thus some care must be given before prescribing any treatment that may restore sexual function in an at-risk patient. The exercise involved in sexual intercourse has been equated to walking up two flights of stairs. It is sometimes necessary to confirm with patients that they are capable of this level of exertion. More precise guidelines have been devised for use before prescribing any ED treatment for a patient with documented cardiac disease (Table 3.3).

TABLE 3.3

Guidelines for prescribing ED treatment in patients with cardiac disease

Risk	Cardiac status	Management
Low	• Controlled hypertension • Mild valvular disease • Mild stable angina • Post revascularization	Manage in primary care
Moderate	• Recent MI or cerebrovascular accident (6 weeks) • Congestive heart failure • Murmur of unknown cause • Moderate stable angina	Specialized evaluation recommended
High	• Uncontrolled angina • Uncontrolled hypertension • Severe heart failure • Recent MI or cerebrovascular accident (2 weeks) • High-risk arrhythmia • Hypertrophic cardiomyopathy • Moderate/severe valve disease	Refer for cardiac opinion

Ocular safety. Several recent reports have suggested a small risk of blindness due to non-arteric anterior ischemic optic neuropathy (NAION) in patients using PDE5 inhibitors. To date, fewer than 50 such cases of NAION have been reported to the US Food and Drug Administration (FDA). Given the large number of men using these agents, it is not possible to determine whether NAION is directly linked to the use of PDE5 inhibitors; however, loss of vision or reduced vision, whether painful or painless, demands urgent patient assessment and immediate cessation of PDE5 inhibitor use.

Sildenafil citrate, the first PDE5 inhibitor for the treatment of ED, has undergone extensive trials involving more than 10 000 men aged 19–87 years and has been used by millions of men throughout the world with ED of organic, psychogenic and mixed etiology. Treatment-related improvements in erections were reported by 70–90% of patients receiving sildenafil versus 10–30% of men receiving placebo. Doses of 50 mg and 100 mg were well tolerated and highly effective in restoring erectile function in flexible-dose studies (Figure 3.2). Study results from more than 550 patients treated for at least 4 years indicate that the efficacy of sildenafil is maintained in the majority of men during long-term treatment (Figure 3.3), although an increased proportion were taking the higher dose of the drug at the study end.

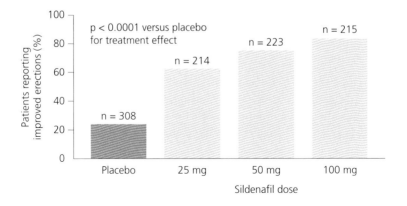

Figure 3.2 Patients treated with sildenafil reported improved erections in clinical trials.

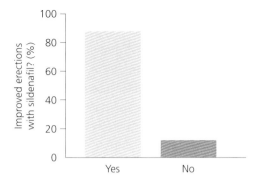

Figure 3.3 After 4 years, most patients still reported improved erections with sildenafil.

Clinical trial data also demonstrate that sildenafil, taken 1 hour before sexual activity, is effective therapy for ED in a wide variety of patients, including those with diabetes (57%), spinal-cord injury (80%), as well as other concomitant medical disorders, such as hypertension (70%) and coronary artery disease (70%). It is effective in patients taking a wide variety of other medications, including antihypertensives and selective serotonin-reuptake inhibitors.

The drug has been shown to help with a number of other domains of sexual function such as orgasmic function, sexual desire, intercourse satisfaction and overall satisfaction. Patients' overall quality of life is enhanced, and partners also experience greater sexual and overall satisfaction rates with men taking sildenafil than those receiving placebo in randomized trials. More recently, studies have indicated that sildenafil treatment can improve self-esteem for men with ED (measured by the Self-Esteem And Relationship questionnaire) and overall confidence levels.

The recommended starting dose of sildenafil is 50 mg taken 30–60 minutes before sexual activity, and ideally on an empty stomach; it should be taken no more than once daily. Based on efficacy and tolerance, the dose may be increased to 100 mg or reduced to 25 mg. Optimal response may require as many as 6 to 8 attempts at the most effective dose. The median time to onset of erection sufficient for penetration is 30 minutes and the duration of action is at least 4 hours.

The adverse events reported in clinical trials with sildenafil were usually transient and mild to moderate in nature. The most commonly reported side effects were headache (16%), flushing (10%), dyspepsia (7%) and nasal congestion (4%). Altered vision, such as temporary and subtle change in color or brightness perception, was also reported in a small number of patients; this effect is dose-dependent and thought to be due to some inhibitory effect of sildenafil on phosphodiesterase type 6, which is present in the photosensory cells of the retina. Adverse effects decline with continued use. No cases of priapism were reported. The overall discontinuation from sildenafil therapy was low – 2.5% compared with 2.3% for those receiving placebo.

Since the launch of sildenafil in 1998, it has become the first-line treatment of choice for most men presenting with ED. Its high efficacy and good safety profile have made it the ideal option for both patients and physicians alike. Not everyone is suitable for this drug, however, and the following patient groups need to consider an alternative therapeutic option:

- patients taking any form of nitrate or nitric oxide donor drug
- patients with retinitis pigmentosa
- patients with a very low libido
- patients with significant cardiac disease (see Table 3.3).

Tadalafil, a highly selective PDE5 inhibitor, has a chemical structure markedly different from that of both sildenafil and vardenafil, and perhaps because of this the drug has slightly different pharmacokinetic properties and in particular a longer half-life and hence duration of action. It has undergone extensive clinical trials in over 6000 subjects. Double-blind placebo-controlled phase II studies showed a dose–response effect and effectiveness in men with ED of varying severity and etiology. Phase III clinical trials included 1112 patients with a mean age of 59 years and with organic, psychological and mixed etiology with mild, moderate or severe ED. The results of pivotal phase III studies are shown in Table 3.4.

The pharmacokinetic characteristics of tadalafil confer certain clinical features. Absorption and activity are not affected by food or alcohol intake, presumably making the dosing regimen more convenient for patients than that of sildenafil. Although the onset of action can be as

TABLE 3.4

Phase III study results for tadalafil versus placebo in various patient groups

Patient response	Placebo	Tadalafil, 20 mg
General:		
Able to complete intercourse satisfactorily?	23%	64%
Improved erections?	19%	79%
Diabetics:		
Able to complete intercourse satisfactorily?	20%	57%
Improved erections?	28%	66%
Men after radical prostatectomy		
Able to complete intercourse satisfactorily?	19%	41%
Improved erections?	23%	62%

short as 16 minutes, optimal treatment response is best achieved (in a typical patient with ED) if the recommended starting dose of tadalafil (20 mg) is taken 1–2 hours or longer before sexual activity. The main difference between tadalafil and the other PDE5 inhibitors, though, is the duration of action of the drug, owing to the prolonged serum half-life of 17.5 hours, which gives a duration of action of over 36 hours. This effect may allow a patient and his partner increased freedom to engage in sexual activity at the time of their choice and thus permit more spontaneous activity by reducing the need to perform within a certain period. At 24 hours following a tadalafil dose of 20 mg, 67% of patients were able to complete intercourse, compared with 42% in the placebo group; at 36 hours, the proportion was 62%, compared with 33% of placebo patients.

Tadalafil was effective in men taking concomitant medications but, like other PDE5 inhibitors, is contraindicated in those taking nitrates. Because of the prolonged half-life of tadalafil, current guidelines suggest that nitrate drugs should not be given for 48 hours after the last dose of tadalafil. Tadalafil appears to have no harmful effects on the cardiovascular system itself, and review of over 4000 patients revealed no reported increases in morbidity or mortality compared with men with ED in the general population. Concomitant administration of tadalafil with non-selective α-blockers can cause hypotension and should be avoided.

Other side effects of tadalafil are mild and transient; in one study, the discontinuation rate due to adverse events was 1.7% (placebo 1.1%). The most common side effects for the 10–20 mg dosages were headache (15%), dyspepsia (10%), back pain (6.5%), myalgia (3%) and nasal congestion (3%). The longer-term safety and tolerability of tadalafil has been demonstrated in open-label extension studies in patients who completed 24 months of treatment.

Tadalafil has relatively little effect on PDE6, so visual disturbance is rare compared with its occurrence with sildenafil. However, it inhibits PDE11, found in skeletal muscle, pituitary tissue and peripheral vascular tissue. Whether this PDE11 inhibition is deleterious or advantageous has yet to be elucidated.

An increasing body of evidence supports the efficacy and safety of chronic daily or alternate-day dosing of tadalafil as a treatment for ED. Daily dosing of tadalafil at doses of 2.5 mg and 5 mg has recently been approved for the treatment of ED in the USA. The evidence suggests that chronic dosing of tadalafil is as, or more, effective than on-demand dosing; this dosing regimen may have a role in the salvage of PDE5 inhibitor non-responders, or as part of a program to rehabilitate erectile function after nerve-sparing radical prostatectomy for prostate cancer.

Vardenafil is a more potent PDE5 inhibitor in vivo than sildenafil or tadalafil, but there is no convincing clinical evidence based on well-designed head-to-head comparator studies to suggest a superior erectile response during home use by men with ED. Once again, this drug has been extensively studied in variable-dose randomized, placebo-controlled trials across a broad range of patient populations with ED. At doses of 10 and 20 mg, 77% of men reported improvement in the quality of their erections after 12 weeks of treatment, compared with 28% taking placebo. Similar improvements have been shown for other domains of sexual function such as orgasmic function, intercourse satisfaction and overall satisfaction, with a mean of 70% successfully completed intercourses in the vardenafil group compared with 25% with placebo. Vardenafil has also been shown to be effective in men with ED of various etiologies and severities and has demonstrated efficacy in traditionally resistant patient populations such as diabetics and men who have undergone radical prostatectomy. Vardenafil has also been shown to be effective in men who had previously failed to respond to sildenafil.

In phase III studies, successful intercourse increased from 32.2% with placebo to more than 66% with 20 mg vardenafil. Phase III studies on sub-groups such as those with diabetes have confirmed the safety and efficacy in these men, while in diabetic patients, improvement in successfully completed intercourse increased from less than 10% at baseline to 54% with 20 mg vardenafil. In patients who had undergone nerve-sparing radical prostatectomy, successful completion of intercourse increased from 10% at baseline and with placebo to 37% with vardenafil treatment. When patients were asked whether their erections had improved, those treated with vardenafil reported an improvement of 72% compared with 13% from placebo. A number of studies have also evaluated the longer-term safety and efficacy of vardenafil and established that a proportion of men (77% with mild ED at baseline and 39% with severe ED at baseline) are able to restore normal erectile function (IIEF domain score > 26) after 6 months' treatment.

Vardenafil is rapidly absorbed from the gastrointestinal tract, giving a fast onset of action: a retrospective pooled data study indicated an effect within 15 minutes of ingestion, while another study showed activity of the drug as early as 10 minutes. Food and alcohol do not significantly affect the absorption of vardenafil, although a high-fat meal can delay the onset of action. The duration of action is about 8 hours.

Adverse events were those expected of a PDE5 inhibitor and included headache (15%), flushing (12%), rhinitis (10%) and dyspepsia (4%) at the higher doses, with less frequency at the lower dose. Like other PDE5 inhibitors, vardenafil should not be used by men for whom sexual activity is inadvisable or by men taking any form of nitrate drug. Likewise, men who are taking an α-blocker should be warned that its hypotensive effect can be exaggerated and the dose of vardenafil should be minimized.

Comparison of PDE5 inhibitors. A multitude of clinical trials have shown similar overall efficacy for the different PDE5 inhibitors. Other studies have suggested that if one particular PDE5 inhibitor is not effective then another may yield success. There are, however, differences between the drugs in terms of pharmacokinetic profiles and thus drug behavior. Food high in fat delays and reduces the absorption of sildenafil and vardenafil, but does not affect the rate or extent of absorption of tadalafil. The mean time to maximum plasma concentration of sildenafil and vardenafil is 1 hour and for tadalafil is 2 hours, while the half-lives of sildenafil and vardenafil are 4–5 hours and that of tadalafil is 17.5 hours. A number of studies have evaluated patient preference, with differing results depending on the populations studied and the method of identifying drug preference. Patients should be made aware of the differences and may express preference, depending on their patterns of sexual activity, their partners' preferences, their beliefs about ED medications and their self-confidence, that is, factors other than just drug efficacy, safety and tolerability.

Apomorphine. Sexual activity often commences with visual, aural and tactile stimuli (pro-erectile stimuli) acting through higher centers within the brain and the CNS. The importance of these central neurohormonal mechanisms to erectile function has made their pathways a target for centrally acting drugs.

Apomorphine is a dopamine-receptor agonist that acts on the dopaminergic receptors in the paraventricular nucleus of the hypothalamus. This area of the brain activates a neural event that coordinates a sequence of signaling that results in a penile erection. The drug therefore acts as a central initiator of an erection by enhancing and coordinating the pro-erectile stimuli, and, like PDE5 inhibitors, requires sexual stimulation to work. Apomorphine sublingual (SL), which is approved only in Europe and New Zealand, has been administered to more than 3000 men in over 75 000 doses. In the initial phase II placebo-controlled studies, men were given 2, 4, 5 or 6 mg of apomorphine SL. Results showed a dose–response effect with two-thirds of patients achieving successful intercourse at the highest dose. In phase

III crossover double-blind studies in men with mild to moderate ED of multiple etiologies and with multiple comorbidities, erections occurred within 10–25 minutes and at the higher dose of 4 mg, erections sufficient for intercourse were achieved on 54% of attempts, compared with 33% for placebo (Figure 3.4). This overall efficacy is lower than that of PDE5 inhibitors, and the duration of action is shorter.

In another study, a 3 mg dose was not significantly different from 4 mg in efficacy, but had a lower incidence of adverse events. The main adverse effects at doses of 2 and 3 mg (compared with placebo) are:

- nausea (7%)
- headache (7%)
- dizziness (4.5%)
- syncope (1%).

No serious adverse events were seen in any of the large clinical trials. Nausea was most often experienced on first dosage of the drug and less commonly thereafter.

Contraindications are similar to those of the PDE5 inhibitors and any ED product, and include recent myocardial infarction, severe unstable angina and heart failure. Unlike PDE5 inhibitors, however, apomorphine can be used by men taking nitrate medications. Precautions should be observed in men with uncontrolled hypertension, or with renal or hepatic failure, or those using nitrates or dopaminergic

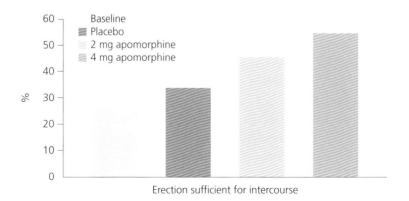

Figure 3.4 Percentage improvement from baseline with apomorphine.

drugs. Patients taking antihypertensive drugs are not affected by coadministration of apomorphine; in a study of 122 men there were no effects on cardiovascular parameters or adverse events.

Yohimbine is derived from the bark of the *Pausinystalin yohimbe* tree which, for over a century, has been thought to possess aphrodisiac qualities. Yohimbine has well-defined properties as an α_2-adrenoceptor-blocking agent, acting both peripherally and centrally. The role of yohimbine in the treatment of ED is more of historic interest; it has been largely replaced by the more effective PDE5 inhibitor drugs. In a small study of men with psychogenic impotence, yohimbine produced a positive response rate of 31% compared with only 5% with placebo; however, in a controlled trial in patients with organic ED, it was found to be no more effective than placebo.

The findings have stimulated research into other α_2-blockers with the potential to produce a better response, and drugs with other actions.

Other novel agents. A number of other oral agents are currently under investigation, mostly new PDE5 inhibitors, as well as cyclic adenosine monophosphate (cAMP) activators, L-arginine and other nitric oxide donors.

Udenafil, a long-acting PDE5 inhibitor, has been approved in South Korea and phase III trials are being conducted in North America, with planned submission for approval by the FDA and other regulatory bodies at some stage in the future.

Nitric oxide, the key neurotransmitter for erectile function, is synthesized from L-arginine by the enzyme nitric oxide synthetase. It appears that L-arginine may not be effective alone, but may have a role in combination with other oral agents.

Despite several clinical trials, there are no convincing data to support the efficacy of natural therapies such as Ginko Biloba extract or Korean Red Ginseng in the treatment of ED.

Vasoactive drug therapy

Intracavernosal and intraurethral vasoactive drug therapy is often useful in men with ED and particularly effective in men with any form of neurogenic dysfunction. These men have a normal hemodynamic mechanism, but lack the control system that initiates the erectile response; this response can, however, be stimulated by any of the vasoactive agents. This observation is true for any of the neurogenic causes of ED including diabetic autonomic neuropathy. Psychogenic ED, which can also be regarded as a failure of appropriate neurotransmission to the erectile tissues, will often also respond very favorably to this treatment.

As experience with these agents has increased, men with other causes of ED have been treated, in particular men with vascular insufficiency, who form the largest group of patients with organic etiologies in an ED clinic. High local concentrations of smooth-muscle relaxant drugs act on both the trabecular muscle and the arteriolar vasculature and are able to overcome mild arterial insufficiency. However, when the arterial supply is severely compromised, pharmacologically induced arterial dilatation is more difficult to achieve because it cannot facilitate sufficient inflow to engorge the lacunar spaces and thereby operate the veno-occlusive mechanism.

Although all vasoactive drugs produce some degree of erectile response when injected directly into the corpus cavernosum, so far only four have found widespread current clinical use: papaverine, phentolamine, prostaglandin E_1 and vasoactive intestinal peptide (VIP). The others have failed to do so because of either lack of efficacy or side effects caused by leakage of the drug into the systemic circulation.

Intracavernosal therapy

The efficacy and safety of self-injection with vasoactive drugs has been demonstrated over the last 20 years. This form of treatment has proved effective in more than 90% of men with other types of erectile disorder and is especially important for men who fail PDE5 inhibitor therapy (Table 3.5).

Papaverine is a powerful direct smooth-muscle relaxant that acts on both the trabecular muscle of the erectile tissue and the vascular tone, inducing an erection that lasts for several hours. When vasoactive agents were introduced, papaverine was initially the most widely used

53

TABLE 3.5

Indications for intracorporal self-injection with vasoactive drugs

Good response
- Psychogenic ED
- Neurogenic ED

Moderate response
- Mild arterial insufficiency
- Mild veno-occlusive disorder
- Drug-induced ED
- Age-related ED
- Diabetes mellitus

Poor response
- Severe arterial insufficiency
- Severe veno-occlusive disorder
- Very elderly men

agent for intracorporal self-injection. It has been extensively studied and shown to be effective. Data from over 4000 men in clinical trials have shown that about 70% of all men who attended an ED clinic obtained an erection sufficient for sexual intercourse. The dose necessary to achieve this can vary from 10 mg to 80 mg, and it is necessary to carefully titrate the dose to achieve a maximal response with minimal risk of priapism. For those men who have failed to get an adequate response from papaverine alone, combination therapy with phentolamine and prostaglandin E_1 (Trimix) may prove beneficial.

Phentolamine acts principally to reduce adrenergically induced vascular smooth-muscle tone, and probably does not initiate an erection very effectively on its own. It is used in combination with papaverine or with papaverine combined with prostaglandin E_1 (Trimix), and appears to work synergistically with it, acting directly on the α-adrenoceptors of the vascular smooth muscle to potentiate the effects of papaverine.

Prostaglandin E_1. In 1913, it was established that an extract of human prostate, called prostaglandin, was able to reduce blood pressure. By 1985, prostaglandin E_1 (alprostadil) had been isolated and shown to cause relaxation of smooth muscle in the corpus cavernosum via an adenylate cyclase cAMP second messenger system. It is a natural body constituent found in high concentrations in the seminal vesicles and corpora cavernosa, and is actively metabolized in the lung (70% first-pass metabolism), liver and kidney. Alprostadil acts by inhibiting α-adrenergic tone in the penile vasculature and by relaxing trabecular smooth muscle.

Recently, alprostadil has become the drug of choice for intracavernous pharmacotherapy. Prostaglandin E_1 plays a role as a neurotransmitter in the natural erectile mechanism, and alprostadil is at least as effective in treating ED as combination therapy with papaverine and phentolamine, and appears to have fewer side effects. As a result, the alprostadil preparations Caverject®, Edex® and Viridal Duo® have been licensed for the treatment of ED in Europe and the USA. There are now data on over 10 000 men with ED who have self-injected with alprostadil. In one study of 550 men, over 70% of patients achieved an erection sufficient for sexual intercourse that lasted for at least 30 minutes and, in another study, 77% of sexual partners reported the erections to be 'good' or 'very good', with 74% reporting an improvement in their relationship. Studies have demonstrated excellent efficacy in patients failing PDE5 inhibitor therapy.

The final therapeutic dose of drug must be titrated up to prevent the risk of priapism, although this risk is considerably less than that with papaverine. The effective dose can range from 5 μg to 20 μg depending on the etiology of the ED. Occasionally, larger doses (up to 60 μg) are required.

Vasoactive intestinal polypeptide is a neurotransmitter that acts on the adenylate cyclase system of the smooth muscle cell, reducing intracellular calcium and initiating relaxation. When used in isolation as an intracavernosal agent, it has a lower efficacy than other injectable agents, but it has been shown to be very effective in combination with phentolamine (Invicorp™). In a study of over 550 men with predominantly organic ED, 83% were able to achieve erections with one of the two doses available. Adverse events were uncommon, with prolonged erections occurring in only 3 men, and pain on injection was rarely reported. Phentolamine–VIP and the injector device are well tolerated by patients and partners alike.

Combination therapy. In men who fail to get an adequate response from papaverine alone, combination therapy with phentolamine, papaverine and prostaglandin E_1 often proves beneficial. Phentolamine, acting directly on the α-adrenoceptors of the vascular smooth muscle, appears to potentiate the effects of papaverine and prostaglandin E_1.

Other vasoactive drugs and drug combinations, such as the combination of phentolamine and VIP, are being introduced, and their therapeutic potential is currently under evaluation. Triple mix, or trimix, consisting of alprostadil, papaverine and phentolamine, is used for difficult-to-treat patients. The vasoactive agents discussed here can also be used in combination with PDE5 inhibitors.

Contraindications. Papaverine, phentolamine and alprostadil have a low rate of leakage into the systemic circulation, resulting in few contraindications to their use. There are, however, some relative contraindications (Table 3.6).

Self-injection technique. Intracavernosal therapy is, in general, used by men who have failed to respond to PDE5 inhibitors in whom the use of PDE5 inhibitors is contraindicated. However, a significant number of men who respond to oral therapy may choose to continue using self-injection on occasions when oral therapy is inconvenient. The self-

TABLE 3.6

Relative contraindications to vasoactive drug therapy

- Sickle-cell trait or disease
- Leukemia
- Anticoagulation
- Poor manual dexterity
- Bloodborne infections, such as HIV or hepatitis
- Previous history of priapism

injection technique should be taught by either the physician or the practice nurse; the tuition should include self-administration of an injection by the patient under direct supervision (Figure 3.5).

With alprostadil, the recommended starting dose is 2.5 mg for patients with known neurogenic or psychogenic impotence, and 5 mg for others, with the dose being doubled on each successive injection. In patients who experience intolerable pain after injection with prostaglandin E_1, or if prostaglandin E_1 is unavailable, papaverine may be used at a starting dose of 5 mg, increasing in 5 mg increments. These recommendations are suitable for patients with suspected neurogenic or psychogenic ED, but if there is known arterial insufficiency, the starting dose is usually higher. When a satisfactory erection is achieved, the patient and his partner will gain confidence with the technique.

First, the patient, or his partner, must become familiar with the handling of the needles and syringes and the technique of drawing up drug solutions. In addition, alprostadil needs to be reconstituted from powder before injection. The skin over the penis is drawn taut, and the

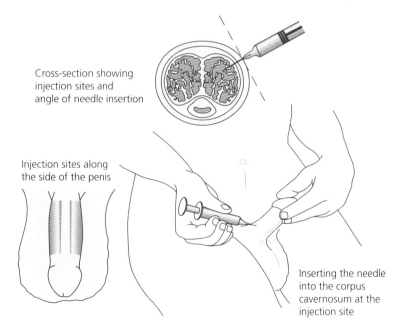

Cross-section showing injection sites and angle of needle insertion

Injection sites along the side of the penis

Inserting the needle into the corpus cavernosum at the injection site

Figure 3.5 Self-injection technique.

needle and syringe held at right angles to the penis (Figure 3.5). The injection is given near to the base of the penis on either side and avoiding any visible veins. Injection sites should be varied and compressed with an alcohol swab for approximately 60 seconds after the injection. Teaching demonstrations, illustrated manuals and videos, all of which are available from the manufacturers, are recommended.

Side effects from self-injection of vasoactive agents (Table 3.7) can be classified as:
- treatment failure
- unwanted local effects
- unwanted vasodilatory systemic effects (e.g. flushing and hypotension).

Treatment failure. The most common side effect is treatment failure: 80% of failures are due to incorrect administration of the drug into the corpora cavernosa, usually as a result of incorrect injection technique. If injections continue to be ineffective despite correct technique, a higher drug dose may be necessary. Systemic side effects are uncommon (about 1%) and result from leakage of the drug into the circulation. Phentolamine has been reported to occasionally cause dizziness, tachycardia and hypotension, as has alprostadil, and papaverine has been associated with occasional derangement of liver function. These observations have not led to any significant limitation in the use of these agents.

TABLE 3.7

Comparison of side effects of injectable agents

	Alprostadil	VIP + phentolamine	Papaverine + phentolamine
Priapism	0.5–1.3%	< 0.5%	2–8%
Pain on injection	17–50%	1%	1%
Hematoma	3%	3%	3%
Systemic effects	1%	10–50%	5–20%

VIP, vasoactive intestinal peptide.

Priapism. The most troublesome side effect with any of these drugs is the development of a prolonged erection, or priapism. Any erection lasting for more than 2 hours should be regarded as a prolonged erection; any erection lasting for 4 hours or more, especially if painful, should be regarded as a priapism and treatment sought. Patients must be warned in advance of this potential complication, both verbally and in writing, and should be given instructions on what they should do in the event of a priapism. The occurrence of priapism is dose-dependent with each of the drugs, and tends to occur during the early stages of titration during a treatment program. The incidence of priapism after injection with alprostadil has been reported to be between 0.5% and 1.3%.

In the event of a prolonged erection, patients should administer pseudoephedrine, 120 mg. Pseudoephedrine is relatively contraindicated in men with hypertension and coronary artery disease. If a priapism occurs, medical intervention should be sought within 6–8 hours.

Failure to achieve detumescence after 6–8 hours can cause irreversible ischemic damage to the corpora cavernosa with subsequent fibrotic damage and permanent loss of erectile function. A priapism is a medical emergency and patients should be referred to an accident and emergency department for treatment.

In most cases, priapism can be relieved by simple aspiration of blood (in 50–100 mL portions) through a needle of appropriate caliber placed in the corpora cavernosa, usually combined with irrigation of the corpora with a dilute vasoconstrictor such as phenylephrine. A small number of patients who fail to respond to detumescence pharmacotherapy may require surgical decompression of their priapism using a variety of shunt procedures.

Other local side effects include the formation of fibrotic nodules around the injection site after repeated use (which can lead to penile curvature), hematoma formation, and diffuse pain along the shaft of the penis immediately after injection. Discomfort in the penile shaft is thought to be more common with the use of prostaglandin E_1 than the other vasoactive drugs, but this does not often result in the cessation of therapy.

Topical intraurethral therapy

A pellet of alprostadil has been developed for insertion into the urethra through a specific polypropylene applicator. Once delivered, the pellet dissolves into the urethral mucosa and from there enters the corpora.

Alprostadil is a synthetic form of prostaglandin E_1; it acts via the adenylate cyclase system to reduce intracellular calcium and induce smooth-muscle relaxation. The administration system is marketed as MUSE® (Medicated Urethral System for Erection; Figure 3.6). Men are asked to urinate before use, as this aids insertion of the applicator and facilitates the intraurethral dispersion of the drug. While in the sitting position, the patient inserts the applicator and then depresses the ejector button, releasing the alprostadil pellet. The penis is then held upright and gently rolled to disperse the drug. Erections develop about 10–15 minutes after application and last for approximately 30 minutes.

Early results with this treatment reported a dose–response effect with 66% of men with ED (all causes) obtaining a full erection, though subsequent studies have reported a lower efficacy. The doses required to achieve this ranged from 125 to 1000 µg. The side effects of this treatment are those of penile pain (7%) and minor urethral trauma

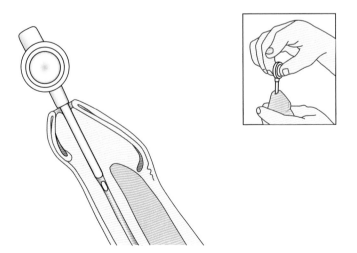

Figure 3.6 Intraurethral administration of alprostadil using the MUSE® system.

(1%). In a comparative study of intracavernosal and intraurethral application of alprostadil, the intracavernosal administration was shown to be more effective though there was a slightly higher incidence of local side effects than with the intraurethral route of administration. It would thus seem that while the intraurethral route of administration is associated with a lower overall success rate, the improved side-effect profile and acceptability to patients may make it a preferred option for some patients. MUSE may also be effective in men with failed penile implants.

A new topical alprostadil preparation is under development that is applied to the glans penis. Early reports suggest effectiveness in as many as 75% of patients with few side effects.

Androgen replacement therapy for hypogonadal men

In men with a proven testosterone deficiency, testosterone replacement therapy can be effective, not only in improving sexual function, but also enhancing well-being and libido. Reliable diagnosis of hypogonadism requires a pool of two or three morning samples to minimize the effect of the diurnal rhythm of testosterone secretion. Approximately 1% of men with ED have hypogonadism but it is unlikely to be present unless the plasma testosterone level is less than 8 nmol/liter. Delivery methods include oral administration, intramuscular injection, skin patches and gels.

All forms of androgen replacement carry the theoretical risk of stimulating prostate growth and promoting the development of latent foci of prostate cancer. Although it is difficult to quantify these risks, and they are probably small, it is important that any patient receiving this treatment is fully informed and his prostate-specific antigen (PSA) level is monitored. Other side effects may include hepatotoxicity, polycythemia, changes in lipids and worsening sleep apnea.

Oral administration. Two types of oral testosterone are available – modified and unmodified. Unmodified testosterone is rapidly absorbed and degraded by the liver, making it difficult to achieve satisfactory serum concentrations. Modified 17-alkyltestosterones, such as methyltestosterone or fluoxymesterone, usually require large doses and multiple daily dose regimens. In addition, these compounds are associated with occasional idiosyncratic hepatotoxicity, even at relatively low doses.

Testosterone undecanoate (Andriol®) is an oral testosterone medication available in Europe, Asia and Canada. Liver toxicity is significantly reduced because it is absorbed through the lymphatics, and the drug appears to be effective although multiple pills must be taken each day to maintain an adequate serum testosterone level because of relatively poor bioavailability.

Intramuscular injection. Testosterone is esterified to yield testosterone enanthate or testosterone cypionate for intramuscular administration to prevent rapid degradation and to render it more soluble in oily vehicles (which carry the drug in muscle tissue). Intramuscular administration was the delivery method of choice until recently, but has a number of significant drawbacks. These include abnormally high initial serum concentrations of testosterone and estradiol, followed by a decline to subnormal levels before the next injection. Testosterone depot therapy has been reported to produce positive and negative fluctuations in libido, erectile function, energy and mood, in parallel with the variations in serum androgen levels. In addition, patients often find deep intramuscular injections painful and dislike the frequent visits to the doctor that are required.

More recently, long-acting depot-intramuscular injections of testosterone undecanoate, administered every 3 months, have produced and maintained serum testosterone levels within the normal adult male range in men with hypogonadism.

Testosterone implants of fused crystalline testosterone are usually inserted subcutaneously in the lower anterior abdominal wall under local anesthesia using a trochar and cannula, and are usually effective for between 3 and 6 months.

Testosterone skin patches. Several forms of testosterone skin patch are now approved (Androderm™, Andropatch™ and Virormone™). In hypogonadal men, daily application of testosterone patches to the back, abdomen, upper arms or thighs produces hormone levels that parallel the endogenous diurnal pattern of serum testosterone characteristic of normal men. Patients report improvements in mood, energy, libido and sexual function to a statistically significant greater extent than seen with placebo. The only side effects are transient local itching, skin irritation and discomfort related to the patch. Another transdermal delivery system (Testoderm™) uses the skin of the scrotum, which allows testosterone to be rapidly absorbed and thus requires only a small patch. The patch adheres gently to the shaved scrotal skin and does not produce skin irritation.

Testosterone gel. 1% testosterone gel (Androgel™, Testim™) is available in 2.5 g and 5 g doses. The gel is applied without a patch once daily

---

Key points – pharmacological treatment

- Phosphodiesterase type 5 (PDE5) inhibitors are effective in approximately 70% of all men with ED, and in these men they work in about 70% of attempts at sexual intercourse.
- PDE5 inhibitors are well tolerated with mild and predictable side effects that are usually transient.
- PDE5 inhibitors are contraindicated if the patient is taking any nitrate drug.
- PDE5 inhibitors differ in their pharmacokinetics, selectivity and molecular structure, the main difference being duration of action (tadalafil having the longest half-life, at over 17 hours).
- Patients must be instructed how to use PDE5 inhibitors and must be aware of their onset of action, duration and interaction with foods.
- Apomorphine appears to be slightly less effective than PDE5 inhibitors but may be faster acting.
- Prostaglandin E_1 remains the treatment of choice for self-injection therapy.
- Intraurethral therapy is less effective than self-injection therapy but is an alternative for men who fail to respond to oral drug treatment.

and has excellent androgen activity with less skin reactivity than skin patches. A daily application enhances serum testosterone levels and normalizes testosterone metabolites; it has minimal dermatological side effects. Because it is applied once daily, early high levels with subsequent falls in serum testosterone concentrations occur in a diurnal pattern. This medication appears to be more physiological than the intramuscular injection or the oral agents.

A new dihydrotestosterone gel is currently undergoing clinical trials and, once approved, this more active form of testosterone may replace other transdermal testosterone preparations.

Alternative therapies

A multitude of therapies have been devised over the centuries to treat ED. Many of these remedies have become confused with aphrodisiacs, which were aimed at increasing sexual desire rather than ability. Alcohol, herbs, citrus fruit and even the cantharis beetle have variously been described to possess powers that reduce ED. In fact, the cantharis beetle contains cantharidinic acid, which can cause an erection but is also nephrotoxic and may lead to priapism and even death. In the last century, monkey testes were transplanted into men to restore erections, and many penile prostheses were devised. The variety of alternative medicines continues to flourish with pheromones, musks, Maca and herbal extracts being readily available. Many of these products contain a number of constituents, sometimes including yohimbine, and therefore some biological activity can be anticipated. The majority, however, have not undergone any form of conventional clinical trial to confirm their safety or efficacy.

Key references

Carson CC, Burnett Al, Levine LA, Nehra A. The efficiency and safety of sildenafil citrate in clinical populations: an update. *Urology* 2002;60:12–27.

Carson CC, Rajfer J, Eardley I et al. The efficacy and safety of tadalafil: an update. *BJU Int* 2004;93: 1276–81.

Derby CA, Mohr BA, Goldstein I et al. Modifiable risk factors and erectile dysfunction: can lifestyle changes modify risk? *Urology* 2000;56:302–6.

Dula E, Bukofzer S; Perdok R, George M. Double-blind, crossover comparison of 3 mg apomorphine SL with placebo and with 4 mg apomorphine SL in male erectile dysfunction. *Eur Urol* 2001;39: 565–70.

Goldstein I, Lue TF, Padma-Nathan H et al. Oral sildenafil in the treatment of erectile dysfunction. *N Engl J Med* 1998;338:1397–404.

Heaton JPW. Key issues from the clinical trials of apomorphine SL. *World J Urol* 2001;19:25–31.

Herrman HC, Chang G, Klugherz BD, Mahoney PD. Hemodynamic effects of sildenafil in men with severe coronary artery disease. *N Engl J Med* 2000;342:1622–6.

Lee LM, Stevenson RW, Szasz G. Prostaglandin E_1 versus phentolamine papaverine for the treatment of erectile impotence: a double-blind comparison. *J Urol* 1989;141:549–50.

Levine SB, Althof SE, Turner LA et al. Side-effects of self-administration of intracavernous papaverine and phentolamine for the treatment of impotence. *J Urol* 1989;141:54–7.

Linet OI, Ogring FG. Efficacy and safety of intracavernosal alprostadil in men with erectile dysfunction. *N Engl J Med* 1996;334:873–7.

Mittelman MA, Glasser DB, Rosazem J. Clinical trials of sildenafil citrate (Viagra) demonstrate no increase of risk of myocardial infarction or cardiovascular death compared with placebo. *Int J Clin Pract* 2003;57:597–600.

Padma-Nathan H, Hellstrom WJG, Kaiser FE et al. Treatment of men with erectile dysfunction with transurethral alprostadil. *N Engl J Med* 1997;336:1–7.

Porst H. Transurethral alprostadil with MUSE vs intracavernous alprostadil – a comparative study in 103 patients with erectile dysfunction. *Int J Impot Res* 1997;9:187–92.

Porst H, Padma-Nathan H, Thibonnier M, Eardley I. Efficacy and safety of vardenafil, a selective phosphodiesterase 5 inhibitor, in men with erectile dysfunction on antihypertensive therapy. *Eur Urol Suppl* 2002;1:152(a593).

Porst H, Rosen R, Padma-Nathan H et al. The efficacy and tolerability of vardenafil, a new, oral, selective phosphodiesterase type 5 inhibitor, in patients with erectile dysfunction. *Int J Impot Res* 2001;13:192–9.

Virag R. Intracavernous injection of papaverine for erectile failure. *Lancet* 1982;ii:938.

The vacuum constriction device is one of the most time-honored methods of treating ED. Its design was first patented in 1917 by Dr Otto Lederer and, although the construction and design of the devices has become more sophisticated, the concept remains the same – a vacuum is applied to the penis for a few minutes, causing tumescence and rigidity, which is sustained using a constricting ring at the base of the penis.

Physiology

The physiological changes that occur in a penis during a vacuum-induced erection are quite different from those that occur during a normal or a pharmacologically induced erection. Trabecular smooth-muscle relaxation does not occur; blood is simply trapped in both the intracorporal and extracorporal compartments of the penis. Distal to the constricting band of the device, venous stasis and decreased arterial inflow lead to penile distension, but also to cyanosis, edema and a progressive drop in skin temperature. Consequently, vacuum-induced erections eventually become uncomfortable and should not be maintained for more than 30 minutes. In addition, the penis only becomes rigid distal to the constricting bands, rather than along the whole corporal length. As a result, the penis tends to pivot inconveniently at its base.

Equipment and technique

Although many different devices are now manufactured, they all have three common components: a vacuum chamber, a pump and a constriction band that is applied to the base of the penis once an erection is achieved (Figure 4.1). The vacuum chamber is made of clear plastic and is open at one end. This is placed over the penis and, with the help of a lubricant jelly, a seal is formed between the chamber and skin, and the pump mechanism then creates a vacuum of at least 100 mmHg, which draws in sufficient blood to create an erection. The

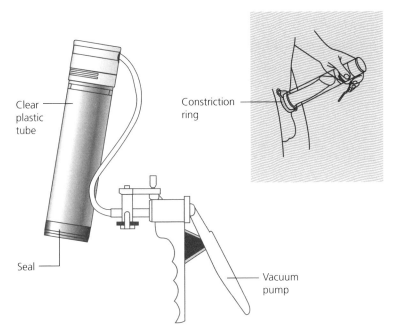

Figure 4.1 A typical vacuum erection device, which is placed over the penis and used to induce an erection that is maintained with a constriction ring.

pump mechanism may be either attached to the vacuum chamber itself or separate from it, and may be either hand or battery operated. Once an erection develops, an elastic ring (the constriction band) is slipped off the chamber to maintain the rigidity by preventing blood escape without injury to the penis. These constriction rings are available in a variety of different sizes.

Clinical use

Because the mechanism of erection is non-physiological, the vacuum constriction device is theoretically suitable for most men who experience ED. Indeed, in one study, 98% of men were able to achieve an erection sufficient for sexual intercourse using one of these devices. In clinical practice, the proportion of men who successfully use this technique is about the same as that who find satisfaction with intracavernosal self-injection. In one report, men who responded well to papaverine were the same group of men who responded well to the vacuum device. As

67

TABLE 4.1

Relative contraindications to the use of vacuum devices

- Sickle-cell trait or disease
- Leukemia
- Anticoagulation, bleeding disorders
- Poor manual dexterity

with self-injection, there are some instances when caution should be observed (Table 4.1).

Side effects

Complications arising from the use of these devices are generally of a minor nature. Petechiae due to capillary rupture are common and transient (10%); hematoma formation is less common (about 5% of patients) and often associated with application of a vacuum pressure that is too high. Other complaints from men using these devices include numbness in the penis (occurring in 75% of users at some stage), a feeling of cold, blue discoloration of the penis and altered or diminished sensation of orgasm (Table 4.2).

Orgasm is often dry, due to the constriction ring which compresses the urethra and so prevents normal ejaculation and often causes some discomfort. Users have also commented on the lack of spontaneity of sexual relations associated with the use of these devices. Despite these complaints, some men do not seem to be deterred from using vacuum

TABLE 4.2

Side effects of vacuum devices

Numbness/coldness in penis	75%
Lack of ejaculation	50%
Altered sensation at orgasm	25%
Hematoma/petechiae	15%
Discomfort on orgasm	9–11%

devices and most studies show a reasonable rate of patient and partner satisfaction (68–83%) with the technique.

Key points – vacuum devices

- A vacuum erection device is an effective treatment option for most etiologies of ED.
- The side effects are prohibitive for some men.
- The treatment does not involve the use of any drugs.

Key references

Bodansky HJ. Treatment of erectile dysfunction using active vacuum assist devices. *Diabetic Med* 1994;11:410–12.

Bosshardt RJ, Farwerk R, Sikora R et al. Objective measurement of the effectiveness, therapeutic success and dynamic mechanisms of the vacuum device. *Br J Urol* 1995;75:786–91.

Nadig PW. Vacuum erection devices. A review. *World J Urol* 1990;8: 114–17.

Wespes E, Schulman CC. Haemodynamic study of the effect of vacuum device on human erection. *Int J Impot Res* 1990;2:337.

Surgical treatment of ED is usually reserved for patients in whom more conservative therapy has failed, or for whom conservative therapy is contraindicated. Most of these patients will have significant arterial or venous disease, penile corpus cavernosum fibrosis or Peyronie's disease, or will, by choice, prefer the prospect of a 'one-off' solution. While the outcome of surgical intervention may be more reliable in certain selected patients, the incidence of morbidity and complications is significantly greater than with medical treatment.

Penile prosthetic implants

Surgically implantable penile prostheses are classified as either semi-rigid or inflatable. Many types with various modifications are widely available. Implants provide penile rigidity and erectile size that adequately simulate the normal physiological erectile state required for sexual intercourse. After careful assessment and discussion with the patient and his partner on their preference, the implants are sized during surgery. The degree of flaccidity differs according to the type of device selected.

Semi-rigid rod prostheses were the first prostheses designed to restore erections and erectile function, and are still used extensively. A variety of semi-rigid rod penile prostheses of different designs are currently available. These prostheses consist of two flexible rods or cylinders that can be varied in length by trimming the proximal portion or adding measured extensions to the proximal portion to fit the patient's measurements (Figure 5.1). Curvature is adjusted via the flexibility provided in their design, which usually includes a central, braided metal wire allowing upward or downward deviation of the prosthesis. Mechanical modifications of these devices include hinges to increase the flexibility and ability to position the prosthesis.

Surgical implantation of these semi-rigid rod prostheses is the simplest type of procedure. A dorsal, subcoronal penile incision, a penoscrotal incision, ventral penile incision, or a perineal incision may

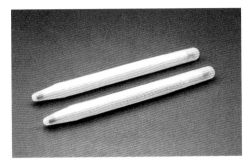

Figure 5.1 Semi-rigid rod penile prostheses are implanted into the corpora cavernosa. They comprise two rods that are trimmed in length intraoperatively, fitted in width and adjusted in curvature through the flexibility provided in their design.

be used to access the corpora cavernosa for dilatation of the corpora and implantation.

Inflatable penile prostheses are available in self-contained, two-piece and three-piece designs (Figures 5.2 and 5.3).

Two-piece inflatable penile prostheses contain two completely inflatable cylinders and a pump/reservoir. This pump/reservoir provides a limited, but usually adequate, volume of fluid for inflation and deflation of the prosthesis. The two-piece design avoids the need for an abdominal fluid reservoir, which is used in three-piece inflatable prostheses. The two-piece design also has an advantage over the self-contained prostheses by increasing the volume of fluid placed in the penile cylinders to improve both erectile inflation and flaccidity. Because of the size of the pump/reservoir, however, flaccidity may not be as complete as with the three-piece inflatable prostheses. Implantation of this device is similar to that described below for the three-piece inflatable penile prosthesis.

Three-piece inflatable penile prostheses are the most complex, yet most cosmetic penile prosthetic devices available. Two inflatable cylinders are placed in the hollow corpora cavernosa and connected to a small pump implanted in the scrotum lateral to the testicle, which is used to inflate and deflate the cylinders, thereby simulating a normal erection. Saline is provided from a reservoir placed beneath the rectus

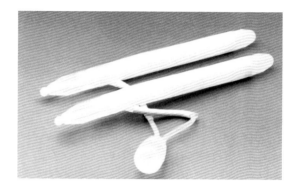

Figure 5.2 A two-piece inflatable prosthesis with a combined pump and reservoir.

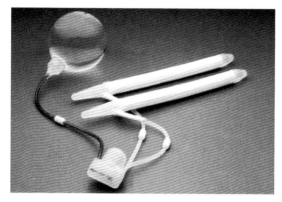

Figure 5.3 A three-piece inflatable implant showing the separate pump, reservoir and cylinders.

muscles of the abdomen. Because of the significant volume provided by this reservoir for both inflation and deflation, both the erect and flaccid states produced are usually excellent. The three-piece inflatable prosthesis provides greater girth and length in comparison to other devices and the more natural flaccid state facilitates the positioning and carriage of the prosthesis under clothing.

Postoperative care

Patients are treated with antibiotics to prevent infection, and an ice pack may be applied to the genitalia after the operation. Oral analgesics are also administered. In addition, with inflatable devices, patients are asked to check the position of the pump for 4–6 weeks before activation to maintain its dependent position in the scrotum. Patients then return to learn how to activate and deflate the device 6 weeks or so after the operation.

Postoperative complications. Although the incidence of postoperative complications has decreased markedly since their introduction, mechanical malfunction can still occur with any of the penile prosthetic devices. The semi-rigid rod penile prostheses may require replacement due to cable fracture or reduced rigidity. Inflatable prostheses are, however, more likely to suffer mechanical complications, although reported mechanical malfunction rates are currently less than 5% over 3 years. Fluid leakage is the most common problem with inflatable prostheses; leaks most commonly occur in the cylinders, which are the portion of the device under the highest pressure. In all cases, device malfunction requires surgical exploration and replacement of the faulty parts of the prosthesis.

Another potential complication is infection; this occurs in 3–5% of patients with older penile prostheses. Higher infection rates can be expected in patients who have had alterations or repairs to their prosthesis, and those with autoimmune diseases and diabetes mellitus. Newer penile implants are coated with antibiotics (InhibiZone) or anti-adherence coatings that absorb and elute antibiotics (the Titan implant). InhibiZone-coated devices have reduced infection rates by more than 60%. The usual procedure for patients with infection is prosthesis removal, healing and subsequent replacement.

Other complications that can arise include erosion of the prosthesis, sustained pain, reduced penile length and reduction in sensation. These complications, though rare, are of significant concern to those men affected and their partners, as well as the surgeon involved.

Patient and partner satisfaction

A number of studies have assessed the outcome and the degree of postoperative satisfaction of patients undergoing penile prosthesis implantation. In general, satisfaction rates are high with all types of implant. The success of surgical treatment is linked to expectations, to the relationship between the patient and his partner and to the preoperative psychological state of the patient. One study comparing satisfaction rates identified no significant difference in patient satisfaction with the semi-rigid and inflatable devices, but when the patients' sexual partners were included in the survey, greater satisfaction with inflatable implants was noted.

Key points – surgical treatment

- Surgery involves dilatation of the erectile tissue of the penis and therefore is a treatment of last resort.
- Penile prostheses have an incidence of infection at insertion and a mechanical failure rate.
- Satisfactory results, for patient and partner alike, can be achieved when other treatments have failed.

Key references

Beutler LE, Scott FB, Karacan I et al. Women's satisfaction with partner's penile implant: inflatable versus noninflatable prosthesis. *Urology* 1984;24:552–8.

Carson CC. Penile prostheses. In: Carson CC, Kirby RS, Goldstein I, eds. *Textbook of Erectile Dysfunction*. Oxford: Isis Medical Media, 1999.

Carson CC, Mulcahy JJ, Govier FE. Efficacy, safety and patient satisfaction outcomes of the AMS 700 CX inflatable penile prosthesis: results of a long-term, multicenter study. *J Urol* 2000;164:628–33.

Steege JF, Stout AL, Carson CC. Patient satisfaction in Scott and Small–Carrion penile implant recipients: a study of 52 patients. *Arch Sex Behav* 1986;15:393–9.

Woodworth BE, Carson CC, Webster GD. Inflatable penile prosthesis: effect of device modification on function longevity. *Urology* 1991;38:533–6.

A number of medical conditions are commonly associated with ED, including:

- depression
- diabetes mellitus
- hypertension
- vascular disease
- endocrine abnormalities.

As noted in Chapter 1, ED may serve as an early indicator for vascular disease.

There are other conditions, described below, that are likewise associated with ED. If primary care physicians are aware of these links, patients with such conditions can be warned of the risk of ED, and early diagnosis and treatment should be possible. Conversely, ED can be a cause of premature ejaculation, which, along with other types of ejaculatory dysfunction, is covered in Chapter 7 (page 81).

Peyronie's disease

Peyronie's disease is curvature of the penis due to fibrosis within the tunica albuginea. The affected corpora cavernosa cannot lengthen on erection, leading to curvature. The condition is most common in middle-aged men who are sexually active. Its exact etiology remains unknown, but it may result from trauma and bleeding into the tunica, followed by activation of the inflammatory process and fibrosis. The more recent observation that HLA class II antigens are more common in men with Peyronie's disease suggests an underlying autoimmune cause. Erectile dysfunction occurs in 30–40% of men with Peyronie's disease. Although the mechanism of their ED is not clearly understood, most appear to have a vascular problem, such as arterial insufficiency where the fibrosis actually distorts the vessels, or failure of the veno-occlusive mechanism.

To a certain extent, treatment is determined by whether the patient has ED and Peyronie's disease. If the patient has this combination, he may be best advised to undergo insertion of a penile implant, as surgical straightening of the penis alone is unlikely to overcome the ED. If penile curvature alone is the factor that precludes intercourse, surgical correction of the curvature by plaque excision and grafting or the Nesbit operation is favored. This latter procedure involves shortening of the contralateral corpus cavernosum. Patients should be warned of the risks of penile shortening and onset of ED after surgery.

Renal failure

Chronic renal impairment is associated with a high incidence of ED, with the incidence increasing with the level of creatinine. Erectile dysfunction is present in about 50% of patients by the time they require dialysis.

A number of factors may be involved, including:

- anemia
- autonomic neuropathy
- reduced testosterone levels with elevated prolactin
- accelerated arterial disease
- other drug therapies
- psychological stress.

After successful transplantation and normalization of renal function, erectile function is restored in many patients. Erythropoietin treatment in patients with renal impairment can also improve the patient's overall quality of life and erectile function.

Pelvic surgery

Any form of pelvic surgery can lead to nerve damage affecting the erectile mechanism. The cavernous nerves run from the pelvic plexus on the lateral border of the rectum down posterolateral to the prostate and into the base of the penis. Damage is, therefore, most likely to occur following surgery to the rectum, bladder or prostate. Improved knowledge of the anatomic course of these nerves has led to the development of nerve-sparing surgical techniques, aided by the Cavermap® nerve stimulation apparatus, that aim to preserve them where possible, but damage cannot be avoided during some operations for malignant disease.

Patients who undergo gastrointestinal surgery that results in an ileostomy or colostomy may suffer depression or loss of self-esteem, which may cause ED. This is particularly relevant to individuals with inflammatory bowel disease requiring excision of the rectum and ileostomy. Patients should always be made aware that specific surgical procedures may lead to ED (Table 6.1). Preliminary evidence suggests that the sooner pharmacological treatment is started after an operation, the more likely the patient is to regain normal erectile function.

Penile injuries

Damage to either the corpora cavernosa or to the neurovascular bundles that supply the corpora can lead to failure of the erectile mechanism.

Corporal injuries. Blunt or penetrating injuries can cause rupture of the tunica albuginea. If not surgically repaired immediately, such injuries can lead to persistent venous leakage through the defect, causing failure of normal corporal filling. The most common cause of blunt trauma is penile fracture (i.e. rupture of the tunica albuginea). This may occur during sexual intercourse or masturbation, and is characterized by an audible crack, followed by penile pain, loss of erection and the onset of a penile hematoma.

Treatment involves urgent exploration and repair of the corporal defect, which should preserve potency in most cases. If repair is delayed for 36 hours or more, ED or penile deformity on erection is a likely consequence.

TABLE 6.1

Risks of ED associated with surgery

Procedure	Reported risks
Radical prostatectomy	10–90%
Radical cystectomy	50–90%
Transurethral resection of the prostate	8%
Anterior resection of rectum	10–50%

Neurovascular bundle injuries. Urethral trauma is the most common cause of injury to the neurovascular bundle, after surgery. It may occur either after a perineal injury and bulbar urethral damage or a pelvic fracture injury and membranous urethral damage. In either instance, it is the neurovascular bundle running posterolateral to the apex of the prostate and posterior urethra that is disrupted. The further the injury is from the membranous urethra, the less likely it is that ED will result. Thus, anterior urethral trauma only occasionally results in this problem.

It has been suggested that prolonged cycling may cause traumatic injury to the pudendal nerves, presumably due to neurovascular compression from the saddle.

Complete urethral disruption injuries from a pelvic fracture are almost universally associated with ED, which may be difficult to treat. Patients often have a combination of both neurological and vascular impairment. Consequently, they do not often respond to conventional pharmacological treatments. In some cases, arterial revascularization surgery should be considered, as this is the subgroup of patients most likely to benefit.

Radiation therapy
Pelvic radiation therapy, whether by external beam or brachytherapy with radioactive seeds inserted into the prostate, can produce ED. While ED rates immediately after external radiotherapy are low – less than 10% at 1 month and 12 months – they increase over time, with 33% of patients reporting ED at 36 months and a mean time to ED of 14.5 months. Similarly, brachytherapy is associated with ED in more than 50% of men 24 months following seed implantation.

Benign prostatic hyperplasia with lower urinary tract symptoms
Recent studies have shown a clear association between ED and benign prostatic hyperplasia with lower urinary tract symptoms. The association is independent of age, but the more severe the lower urinary tract symptoms the more severe the ED. This association is true in all

decades beginning at age 50 through age 70. Recent data have not only confirmed this association but also demonstrated a moderate effect of sildenafil on patients with lower urinary tract symptoms. Because α-blockers are first-line therapy for benign prostatic hyperplasia with lower urinary tract symptoms and preserve erectile function, they may be useful for treating lower urinary tract symptoms and improving ED. However, the US Food and Drug Administration package inserts list a warning for α-blockers taken within 4 hours of sildenafil, permit only tamsulosin in combination with tadalafil, and contraindicate all α-blockers with vardenafil. While sexual dysfunction can occur with the administration of the α-blocker tamsulosin, usually associated with retrograde anejaculation, alfuzosin appears to be effective in treating benign prostatic hyperplasia with lower urinary tract symptoms with fewer sexual side effects.

Ejaculatory dysfunction

Epidemiological studies have suggested that ejaculatory dysfunction, whether retarded ejaculation or premature ejaculation, is as common and as bothersome as ED. Ejaculatory dysfunction affects patients in younger age groups as well as those over 60 years of age. Causes include:

- aging
- low testosterone
- selective serotonin-reuptake inhibitor (SSRI) antidepressants
- pelvic surgery
- psychogenic causes.

While treatments for delayed ejaculation remain elusive and only patients with documented hypogonadism can be improved medically, premature ejaculation can be effectively treated. The original ineffective psychological treatment alternatives have been supplanted by medical treatment. SSRI antidepressants, which may cause objectionable retarded ejaculation in patients receiving high doses, may be used effectively for the treatment of premature ejaculation. Agents such as fluoxetine, paroxetine and sertraline are currently among the agents effective for this treatment. Newer, short-acting on-demand SSRIs are in late-phase trials for the treatment of premature ejaculation; in particular, dapoxetine has undergone extensive phase III trials.

Statistically significant effectiveness versus placebo was demonstrated by
increases in intravaginal ejaculatory latency time as well as by patient
and partner report. Finally, phosphodiesterase type 5 inhibitors may also
be helpful in some patients with mild premature ejaculation. Ejaculatory
dysfunction is discussed in greater detail in Chapter 7.

Key points – associated medical conditions

- Depression, diabetes mellitus, hypertension and vascular disease
  are commonly associated with ED.
- Other conditions and interventions also associated with ED are
  Peyronie's disease, renal failure, pelvic surgery, penile injuries,
  radiation therapy and benign prostatic hyperplasia with lower
  urinary tract symptoms.
- Patients with these conditions should be warned of the risk
  of ED.
- Treatment is often possible.
- Ejaculatory dysfunction is as common and as bothersome as ED;
  treatments are available for premature ejaculation.

Key references

Laumann EO, Paik AM, Rosen RC.
Sexual dysfunction in the United
States: prevalence and predictors.
JAMA 1999;281:527–46.

Rosen R, Altwein J, Boyle P et al.
Lower urinary tract symptoms and
male sexual dysfunction: the
multinational survey of the aging
male (MSAM-7). *Eur Urol*
2003;44:637–49.

Sairam K, Kulinskaya E, McNicholas
TA et al. Sildenafil influences lower
urinary tract symptoms. *BJU Int*
2002;90:836–9.

Ejaculation is a reflex comprising sensory receptors and areas, afferent pathways, cerebral sensory areas, cerebral motor centers, spinal motor centers and efferent pathways. Ejaculatory dysfunction (EjD) is one of the most common male sexual disorders. The spectrum of EjD extends from premature ejaculation (PE), through delayed ejaculation, to a complete inability to ejaculate (anejaculation), and includes retrograde ejaculation and painful ejaculation.

Premature ejaculation

Although approximately 25% of men self-diagnose PE, many of these men experience coincidental and situational rapid ejaculation as a variation of normal ejaculatory function or are overly concerned with a false perception of rapid ejaculation. A recent stopwatch multinational study of a random heterosexual population demonstrated a median intravaginal ejaculation latency time (IELT) of 5.4 minutes and proposed that men with an IELT of less than 1 minute have 'definite' PE. This is consistent with the report that approximately 90% of men who actively seek treatment have an IELT of less than 1 minute. The incidence of PE with an IELT of less than 1 minute is not known.

The International Society of Sexual Medicine (ISSM), using the constructs of time to ejaculation, inability to delay ejaculation and the negative psychological consequences, recently developed a contemporary, evidence-based definition of PE (Table 7.1).

Classification. PE is classified as either lifelong or acquired. Lifelong PE is characterized by early ejaculation, usually within 1 minute in most cases, but occasionally between 1 and 2 minutes, with every, or nearly every, sexual partner, and occurs from the first sexual encounter. Acquired PE is the development of early ejaculation at some point in the individual's life, having previously had normal ejaculation.

Limited correlational evidence suggests that lifelong PE is a genetically determined biological variable related to the inherited

TABLE 7.1

ISSM definition of premature ejaculation

Premature ejaculation is a male sexual dysfunction characterized by:

- ejaculation that always, or nearly always, occurs before or within about 1 minute of vaginal penetration
- the inability to delay ejaculation on all, or nearly all, vaginal penetrations
- negative personal consequences, such as distress, bother, frustration and/or the avoidance of sexual intimacy

ISSM, International Society of Sexual Medicine.

sensitivity of central serotonin (5-HT) receptors, while acquired PE is due to high levels of sexual performance anxiety, ED, prostatitis or thyroid dysfunction.

Management

Lifelong PE is best treated with daily administration of selective serotonin-reuptake inhibitors (SSRIs):

- paroxetine, 20–40 mg
- clomipramine, 10–50 mg
- sertraline, 50–100 mg
- fluoxetine, 20–40 mg.

Paroxetine appears to exert the strongest ejaculation delay, increasing IELT by approximately 8.8-fold from baseline. Ejaculation delay usually occurs within 5–10 days but may occur earlier. Adverse effects are usually minor and start in the first week of treatment, gradually disappearing within 2–3 weeks. They include fatigue, yawning, mild nausea, loose stools and perspiration. Diminished libido or mild ED are infrequently reported. Significant agitation is reported by a small number of patients; treatment with SSRIs should be avoided in men with a history of bipolar depression.

On-demand administration of the drugs listed above 4–6 hours before intercourse is efficacious and well tolerated and is associated with less ejaculatory delay than daily treatment. A number of rapid-acting SSRIs with a short half-life (e.g. dapoxetine) are under investigation as on-demand treatments for PE and are currently under regulatory review by several health authorities. In phase III randomized controlled trials, dapoxetine, 30–60 mg, increased baseline IELT by 3–4-fold, and was well tolerated, with a 20% incidence of nausea (at a dose of 60 mg).

The use of topical local anesthetics such as lidocaine and/or prilocaine is moderately effective in retarding ejaculation. Intracavernous self-injection to treat PE has been reported but there is no evidence-based support for the efficacy of this strategy and it cannot be recommended. There is no empirical evidence to support the efficacy of phosphodiesterase type 5 (PDE5) inhibitors in the treatment of PE except in men with PE and comorbid ED.

Acquired PE due to sexual performance anxiety may be treated with drug therapy, cognitive behavioral therapy (CBT), using techniques such as the 'stop-start' maneuver or the squeeze technique or a combination of both.

Retrograde ejaculation

Retrograde ejaculation, in which ejaculate that would normally exit via the urethra is redirected towards the urinary bladder, is due to bladder neck incompetence. It invariably occurs after transurethral resection of the prostate, and may occur in diabetic autonomic neuropathy or following abdominal aortic aneurysmectomy or para-aortic lymphadenectomy. These men may also have some antegrade ejaculation and usually experience orgasmic sensation.

Retrograde ejaculation can be diagnosed by examining a urine sample, taken after masturbation, for the presence of more than 5–10 spermatozoa per high-power field. Bladder neck reconstruction or drug treatment with sympathomimetic agents such as pseudoephedrine and phenylpropanolamine, or the tricyclic antidepressant imipramine, have produced mixed results. Pregnancy can be achieved using sperm retrieval and artificial insemination techniques.

Delayed ejaculation/anejaculation

Causes of failed emission or delayed ejaculation include spinal trauma, diabetic autonomic neuropathy and surgical procedures such as radical prostatectomy, proctocolectomy, abdominal aortic aneurysmectomy or para-aortic lymphadenectomy. Drug treatment has mixed results.

The ability to ejaculate is severely impaired by spinal-cord injury where, contrary to erectile function, the ability to ejaculate increases with descending levels of spinal injury and completeness of injury. Almost all men with incomplete lower motor-neuron lesions will retain the ability to ejaculate. Pregnancy can be achieved using sperm retrieval techniques such as vibratory stimulation or electroejaculation, which may be complicated by autonomic dysreflexia and severe hypertension.

Inhibited ejaculation is the psychogenic variant of delayed ejaculation. Ejaculation usually occurs readily with solitary masturbation but not during intercourse. A wide variety of psychological factors may be responsible for the inhibition, including fear of pregnancy, religion, guilt, and depressed or repressed hostility towards the partner. Treatment often involves long-term psychotherapy.

Painful ejaculation

Painful ejaculation can be caused by any acute genitourinary infection, particularly acute prostatitis or seminal vesiculitis. It may also have a psychogenic basis. The former can be treated with antibiotics, non-steroidal anti-inflammatory agents, prostatic decongestants such as bromhexine and, if indicated, prostate massage. The latter can be treated by sex therapy.

Key points – ejaculatory dysfunction

- Ejaculatory dysfunction is one of the most common male sexual disorders.
- Men with an intravaginal ejaculatory latency time of less than 1 minute have 'definite' premature ejaculation (PE).
- Lifelong PE, which is genetically determined, is best treated with daily administration of selective serotonin-reuptake inhibitors.
- Acquired PE, due to sexual performance anxiety, may be treated with drug therapy or cognitive behavioral therapy.
- More than 5–10 spermatozoa per high-power field in a postmasturbation urine sample indicates retrograde ejaculation.
- Painful ejaculation can be caused by any acute genitourinary infection, which can be treated with the appropriate drugs, or it may have a psychogenic basis, which will require sex therapy.

Useful resources

UK

British Society for Sexual Medicine
Holly Cottage, Fisherwick
Near Lichfield, Staffs WS14 9JL
Tel: +44 (0)1543 432757/432622
admin@bssm.org.uk
www.bssm.org.uk

British Association of Urological Surgeons
35–43 Lincoln's Inn Fields
London WC2A 3PE
Tel: +44 (0)20 7869 6950
admin@baus.org.uk
www.baus.org.uk

British Urological Foundation
40 Pentonville Road
London N1 9HF
Tel: +44 (0)20 7713 9538
info@buf.org.uk
www.buf.org.uk

Sexual Dysfunction Association
Suite 301, Emblem House
London Bridge Hospital
27 Tooley Street
London SE1 2PR
Helpline: 0870 774 3571
(Mon, Wed, Fri 10 AM–4 PM)
info@sda.uk.net
www.sda.uk.net

USA

American Association of Sexuality Educators, Counselors and Therapists
PO Box 1960
Ashland, Virginia 23005-1960
Tel: +1 804 752 0026
aaset@aaset.org
www.aaset.org

American Urological Association
1000 Corporate Boulevard
Linthicum, MD 21090
Toll-free: 1 866 746 4282
Tel: +1 410 689 3700
aua@auanet.org
www.aua.net.org
www.urologyhealth.org

Center for Urological Care
80 East 69th Street
New York, NY 10021
Tel: +1 212 535 6690
info@urologicalcare.com
www.urologicalcare.com

Consortium for Improvement in Erectile Function
c/o Cognimed Inc
70 South Orange Avenue
Suite 200, Livingston, NJ 07039
Toll-free: 1 800 720 7779
http://erectilefunction.org

International European
Association of Urology
PO Box 30016
NL-6803 AA Arnhem
The Netherlands
Tel: +31 (0)26 389 0680
eau@uroweb.org
www.uroweb.org

International Society for Sexual
Medicine
PO Box 97, 3950 AB Maarn
The Netherlands
Tel: +31 343 443 888
secretariat@issm.info
www.issm.info

Other websites
www.embarrassingproblems.com

www.erectionadvice.co.uk

http://kidney.niddk.nih.gov/
kudiseases/topics/erectile.asp

www.medicinenet.com/impotence_
ed/article.htm

www.nlm.nih.gov/medlineplus/
erectiledysfunction.html

www.sexual-dysfunction.co.uk/
erectile-dysfunction.html

Index

ED stands for erectile dysfunction and EjD stands for ejaculatory dysfunction.

Fast Facts

the ultimate medical handbook series

70 key topics authored by 150 world experts

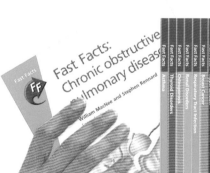

What the reviewers say:

A useful addition to this well-known series . . . very affordable and excellent value for money

On *Fast Facts – Bladder Disorders*, in *ICS News*, Feb 2008

An excellent introduction to minor surgery for the healthcare professional

British Dermatological Nursing Group, on *Fast Facts – Minor Surgery*, 2nd edn, Jan 2008

A clear, concise, easy to read and beautifully illustrated text. I am not lending my copy to anyone!

Professor Stephen R Durham, President, British Society for Allergy & Clinical Immunology, on *Fast Facts – Rhinitis*, 2nd edn, Sep 2007

This splendid book shows a lot of originality ... an excellent, well-structured resource for all healthcare professionals

Mary Baker MBE, Patron, European Parkinson's Disease Association, on *Fast Facts – Parkinson's Disease*, 2nd edn, Apr 2007

I strongly recommend this book as a resource for the busy healthcare professional, both during their training and in practice

On *Fast Facts – Diseases of the Pancreas and Biliary Tract*, in *Can J Gastroenterol* 21(3), 2007

Contains very well-constructed tables and boxes which highlight salient points of diagnosis and management and ... a great many tips on how best to manage patients

Dr Simon Barton, President, British Association for Sexual Health & HIV, on *Fast Facts – Sexually Transmitted Infections*, Feb 2007